NEXT GENERATION NCLEX-PN®

EXAM PREP 2025-2026

MASTER SCORE PUBLICATIONS

Book formatting and cover designed by thiwwy design

Table of Contents

Introduction

Passing the NCLEX-PN is the final step to becoming a Licensed Practical Nurse (LPN), and this book is designed to guide you through every topic tested on the exam with clarity and confidence. The NCLEX-PN follows a structured content framework, assessing your knowledge across key areas of patient care. These include **Coordinated Care (18%-24%), Safety and Infection Control (10%-16%), Health Promotion and Maintenance (6%-12%), Psychosocial Integrity (9%-15%), Basic Care and Comfort (7%-13%), Pharmacological Therapies (10%-16%), Reduction of Risk Potential (9%-15%)**, and **Physiological Adaptation (7%-13%)**. This book is organized to reflect these categories, ensuring a logical progression that aligns with the official NCLEX-PN blueprint.

The **Next Generation NCLEX-PN (NGN)**, introduced in April 2023, brings a stronger emphasis on **clinical judgment, critical thinking, and real-world nursing scenarios.** Unlike previous versions of the exam, the NGN features new question formats designed to assess decision-making skills in **high-pressure, real-life nursing situations.** These include **case studies, matrix multiple-choice, drag-and-drop ordering, and bowtie questions**, all aimed at evaluating how well candidates can apply their nursing knowledge in practice.

This book is fully updated to reflect these **new testing standards**, ensuring that you are well-prepared for every aspect of the NGN exam. Each chapter goes beyond just memorization by focusing on **clinical reasoning, patient care decision-making, and practical nursing applications.** You'll find real-world patient scenarios that mirror the NCLEX experience, along with practice questions designed to help you develop **strong clinical judgment and problem-solving skills.**

Whether you're reviewing fundamental nursing concepts, reinforcing pharmacology knowledge, or strengthening your ability to think critically in a clinical setting, this book provides a **comprehensive yet streamlined approach** to help you succeed on exam day. By studying with this guide, you'll gain the confidence and expertise needed to **pass the NCLEX-PN on your first attempt and step into your role as a skilled and competent LPN.**

ACCESSING YOUR ONLINE STUDY RESOURCES

To help you maximize your NCLEX-PN preparation, this book includes access to additional online study tools. These resources include **interactive flashcards, real-case scenarios, and an online testing tool** designed to reinforce key concepts and enhance your clinical judgment skills.

To access these materials, refer to the **"Access NCLEX-PN Online Resources"** chapter at the end of this book, where you'll find step-by-step instructions for unlocking your study tools. These resources provide practical application opportunities to complement the material covered in this guide, helping you solidify your understanding and prepare with confidence for exam day.

Chapter 1
Coordinated Care

This chapter focuses on the principles and practices of teamwork, communication, and leadership in nursing. It explores how nurses collaborate with interdisciplinary teams, advocate for clients, and utilize resources to achieve optimal outcomes. From delegating tasks to prioritizing care, the strategies outlined here equip nurses to manage complex situations with confidence and efficiency. By mastering coordinated care, nurses can enhance client satisfaction, promote safety, and contribute to a cohesive healthcare environment.

1.1 Guiding Patients Through Healthcare Directives

Healthcare directives are legal documents that enable individuals to communicate their medical preferences in situations where they may no longer be able to voice their wishes directly. These documents ensure that a person's choices regarding treatments and interventions, such as cardiopulmonary resuscitation (CPR), life-sustaining measures, and end-of-life care, are honored and respected. Common types of healthcare directives include advance directives, living wills, and durable power of attorney for healthcare. Each serves a specific purpose but collectively work to safeguard a patient's autonomy in medical decision-making.

The significance of healthcare directives lies in their ability to uphold patient autonomy, a fundamental principle of ethical healthcare. They empower individuals to maintain control over their care, even in challenging circumstances, such as during unconsciousness or severe illness. By clearly documenting a patient's preferences, healthcare directives also reduce uncertainty for families and healthcare providers, ensuring that care aligns with the patient's values and beliefs. This fosters a patient-centered approach, allowing for decisions that reflect personal priorities rather than defaulting to aggressive or unwanted interventions.

1.1.1 Types of Healthcare Directives

Advance Directives: Definition and Purpose

Advance directives are written instructions that outline a person's preferences for medical care in the event they are unable to communicate their decisions directly. These directives provide a framework for healthcare providers and loved ones to follow, ensuring that medical interventions align with the individual's wishes. The primary purpose of advance directives is to protect patient autonomy and prevent confusion or disputes during critical moments. They act as a proactive measure, giving patients a voice in their care, even when they cannot actively participate in decision-making.

Living Wills: Definition, Scope, and Examples

A living will is a type of advance directive that specifically addresses a patient's preferences regarding life-sustaining treatments and interventions. This document comes into effect when an individual is terminally ill, in a persistent vegetative state, or otherwise incapacitated. A living will provides clear guidance on whether to proceed with procedures such as:

- Cardiopulmonary resuscitation (CPR).
- Mechanical ventilation.
- Artificial nutrition and hydration (e.g., feeding tubes).
- Dialysis or other life-prolonging measures.

For example, a living will might state that a patient wishes to forgo artificial ventilation but would accept palliative care to manage discomfort. This document ensures that healthcare providers and family members can act confidently, knowing they are honoring the patient's explicit instructions.

Durable Power of Attorney for Healthcare: Definition, Role, and Examples

A durable power of attorney for healthcare (DPOA-HC), sometimes referred to as a healthcare proxy, is a legal document that designates an individual (the agent) to make medical decisions on behalf of the patient if they are unable to do so themselves. Unlike a living will, which specifies particular treatments, a DPOA-HC grants the agent the authority to interpret the patient's wishes and make decisions in a variety of scenarios.

The role of the DPOA-HC is especially critical when unexpected circumstances arise that are not explicitly covered in a living will. For instance, if a patient is incapacitated due to a traumatic injury and the situation requires immediate decisions about surgical interventions, the agent can step in and make informed choices consistent with the patient's known values and preferences.

By appointing a trusted individual, patients ensure that someone who understands their beliefs and priorities can advocate for their best interests, providing a flexible and responsive approach to decision-making.

1.1.2 Role of Healthcare Directives in Clinical Practice

Healthcare directives play a vital role in recording and communicating patients' medical preferences, providing clarity and guidance for healthcare teams during critical and often emotionally charged situations. They serve as legally binding documents that reflect the patient's wishes regarding specific interventions and overall care, ensuring that their autonomy is respected and upheld throughout the healthcare process.

Recording Patients' Wishes for Cardiopulmonary Resuscitation (CPR)

Healthcare directives allow patients to specify whether they would like to receive CPR in the event of cardiac or respiratory arrest. Some patients may choose to decline CPR due to personal values, the invasiveness of the procedure, or concerns about the quality of life following resuscitation efforts. For example, an advance directive may include a "Do Not Resuscitate" (DNR) order to clearly communicate the patient's decision, guiding the healthcare team to avoid initiating CPR if the patient's heart stops. This prevents unwanted interventions and aligns care with the patient's preferences.

Recording Preferences for Life-Sustaining Treatments

Healthcare directives also address the use of life-sustaining treatments, such as mechanical ventilators or artificial nutrition and hydration. These treatments are critical in preserving life during severe illnesses or injuries but may not always align with a patient's wishes, particularly if recovery is unlikely or the intervention may prolong suffering. For instance, a living will might state that the patient declines long-term mechanical ventilation or feeding tubes but consents to short-term measures aimed at reversible conditions. This ensures the care provided reflects the patient's values and goals.

Guiding End-of-Life Care Decisions

For patients nearing the end of life, healthcare directives outline preferences for comfort measures, palliative care, and other interventions that focus on quality rather than the prolongation of life. Patients may request pain management and emotional support while forgoing aggressive treatments such as chemotherapy or dialysis. These directives help healthcare providers and families navigate sensitive decisions, ensuring that end-of-life care respects the patient's dignity and personal beliefs.

The Legal and Ethical Importance of Honoring Healthcare Directives

Honoring healthcare directives is not only a legal obligation but also an ethical imperative in clinical practice. These documents represent the patient's voice, ensuring that their autonomy is preserved even when they are unable to advocate for themselves. Ignoring or overriding a directive can lead to legal consequences, erode trust in the healthcare system, and cause significant emotional distress for the patient's loved ones.

From a professional ethics perspective, following healthcare directives aligns with the principles of respect for autonomy, beneficence, and non-maleficence. For instance, adhering to a DNR order respects the patient's informed decision to avoid resuscitation, minimizing unnecessary suffering and upholding their dignity. Healthcare providers are tasked with carefully reviewing and implementing these directives to ensure patient-centered care, balancing medical expertise with the patient's expressed values and choices.

1.1.3 Nurse's Role in Healthcare Directives

Nurses play a critical role in supporting patients and families through the process of understanding, creating, and implementing healthcare directives. Their expertise in communication, patient advocacy, and education ensures that directives are both accurately established and respected within clinical settings.

The nurse's role begins with education, ensuring that patients and families are well-informed about healthcare directives and their significance.

- **Importance of Clear Communication:** Nurses serve as a bridge between patients, families, and healthcare providers, fostering open conversations about the purpose and benefits of healthcare directives. Clear communication helps dispel misconceptions, such as the belief that directives only apply to terminally ill patients, and encourages proactive planning for future healthcare needs.
- **Explaining Options and Ensuring Understanding:** Nurses guide patients and families through the different types of healthcare directives, such as living wills, advance directives, and durable power of attorney for healthcare. They explain the purpose of each document, what it covers, and how it aligns with the patient's values and preferences. For instance, a nurse might help a patient understand the implications of a Do Not Resuscitate (DNR) order or the responsibilities associated with appointing a healthcare proxy. By ensuring understanding, nurses empower patients to make informed decisions.

Nurses assist patients in initiating and maintaining their healthcare directives. They often provide resources, such as templates or guidance on state-specific legal requirements, and help clarify medical terminology that might seem overwhelming.

- **Creating Directives:** Nurses can facilitate discussions between patients, their families, and their care team to ensure that the patient's wishes are accurately documented. For example, a nurse might help a patient articulate preferences regarding life-sustaining treatments after a discussion about the potential outcomes of ventilator use.
- **Updating Directives:** Patients' wishes may evolve over time due to changing health conditions, life circumstances, or new medical advancements. Nurses play a key role in encouraging patients to revisit and update their directives as needed to ensure that they remain relevant and reflective of their current goals.

Once healthcare directives are in place, nurses are responsible for ensuring that they are honored during clinical care. This involves:

- **Verifying Directives:** Nurses review the patient's records to confirm the presence of healthcare directives and communicate these preferences to the broader care team.
- **Coordinating Care:** Nurses work closely with other healthcare professionals to ensure that the care provided aligns with the patient's documented choices, such as avoiding unwanted resuscitation efforts or initiating palliative care.

1.1.4 Healthcare Proxies and Surrogacies

A healthcare proxy and a durable power of attorney for healthcare (DPOA-HC) are both tools used to designate a person to make medical decisions on behalf of a patient. However, there are key differences in their scope and application:

- **Healthcare Proxy:** A healthcare proxy is a specific individual appointed to make medical decisions for a patient when they are incapacitated. Their authority is typically limited to healthcare decisions and does not extend to financial or legal matters.
- **Durable Power of Attorney for Healthcare:** A DPOA-HC can have a broader role, depending on how the document is drafted. While its primary function is to authorize healthcare decision-making, it may also include authority over related matters, such as accessing health records or coordinating care with multiple providers.

For example, a healthcare proxy may be appointed to decide whether to proceed with a surgical procedure, while a DPOA-HC might also handle insurance-related communications or review medical bills.

A healthcare surrogate is a person designated to make medical decisions for a patient when no formal healthcare proxy or DPOA-HC has been appointed. Surrogacies are typically established under state laws that prioritize close family members, such as spouses, adult children, or siblings, to serve as the decision-maker.

Healthcare surrogacies are often applied in emergency situations where immediate decisions are required, and the patient has not provided prior directives. For instance, if a patient is admitted to the emergency room unconscious and without any documented directives, the attending physician may consult the patient's spouse or next of kin to make urgent decisions about care.

Examples of Scenarios

- **Proxy vs. Surrogacy in a Clinical Setting:** A patient with a healthcare proxy may require a critical decision about starting dialysis. The healthcare proxy is consulted to determine the appropriate course of action. In contrast, for a patient without directives, their spouse might be identified as a surrogate under state law to decide whether dialysis aligns with the patient's presumed wishes.

- **Addressing Disagreements Between Proxies and Family Members:** Family conflicts may arise when a healthcare proxy's decisions are questioned by other relatives. For example, a healthcare proxy may follow the patient's documented wish to forgo life-sustaining treatments, but a sibling may demand that all possible measures be taken. In such cases, the nurse's role includes mediating discussions, ensuring the proxy has the support and information needed to uphold the patient's choices, and involving ethical committees or legal advisors as necessary.

1.1.5 Scenarios and Practical Examples

Example 1: A Patient with a Living Will Declining CPR

Mr. Thompson, a 78-year-old patient with a terminal illness, has a living will that explicitly states he does not want cardiopulmonary resuscitation (CPR) if his heart stops. During a routine hospital stay, he experiences cardiac arrest. The nurse, upon reviewing his documented living will, immediately communicates the DNR (Do Not Resuscitate) order to the medical team. Instead of initiating CPR, the team focuses on providing comfort measures and supporting his family during this difficult time. This scenario highlights how a living will guides healthcare providers in honoring the patient's end-of-life preferences while preventing unnecessary interventions.

Example 2: Durable Power of Attorney Making Decisions for an Incapacitated Patient

Mrs. Patel, a 65-year-old patient, suffers a severe stroke that leaves her unable to communicate or make decisions. Her durable power of attorney for healthcare, her adult son Ravi, is contacted by the care team. Ravi reviews his mother's advance directive, which indicates her preference to decline mechanical ventilation if there is little chance of recovery. Guided by this information, Ravi makes the decision to forgo invasive life-sustaining measures and instead consents to palliative care. This example illustrates the importance of the DPOA-HC in ensuring decisions reflect the patient's values and documented wishes.

Example 3: Resolving Family Conflicts Regarding a Healthcare Surrogate's Decisions

Mr. Alvarez, a 58-year-old patient without a formal advance directive, is admitted to the ICU in a coma after a car accident. According to state law, his wife Maria is identified as his healthcare surrogate. Maria decides to decline a high-risk surgery based on conversations she had with her husband about his fears of prolonged suffering. However, Mr. Alvarez's adult daughter from a previous marriage strongly disagrees and demands the surgery proceed. The nurse facilitates a family meeting, explaining the role of the surrogate and the ethical obligation to honor the patient's presumed wishes. With additional support from the hospital's ethics committee, the conflict is resolved, and the medical team follows Maria's decision. This scenario underscores the nurse's role in mediating disputes and ensuring patient-centered care.

1.2 Supporting Patient Rights and Advocacy

Patient rights in healthcare settings refer to the fundamental principles that protect individuals' autonomy, dignity, and access to safe and respectful medical care. These rights include the ability to make informed decisions about one's treatment, the right to privacy and confidentiality, and the right to receive equitable care regardless of socioeconomic or cultural background.

Nurses act as intermediaries, bridging the gap between patients and the healthcare system, especially for those who are vulnerable, marginalized, or unable to speak for themselves. By championing patient rights, nurses not only uphold the ethical principles of autonomy and justice but also contribute to improved health outcomes and a more inclusive healthcare environment.

1.2.1 Key Areas of Patient Advocacy

Informed Consent

Informed consent ensures patients understand their treatment options and can make decisions that suit their preferences. Nurses simplify medical terms, explain risks and benefits, and address concerns to help patients make informed choices. For example, a nurse might clarify the side effects of chemotherapy, ensuring the patient fully understands before consenting.

Privacy and Confidentiality

The right to privacy and confidentiality is a fundamental patient right, enshrined in regulations such as the Health Insurance Portability and Accountability Act (HIPAA). Nurses are responsible for safeguarding this right by ensuring that sensitive health information is protected from unauthorized access or disclosure. Advocacy in this area includes preventing breaches, such as discussing a patient's condition in public spaces, and educating patients about their rights to control who can access their medical records. For example, a nurse might intervene if a colleague inadvertently shares patient information inappropriately, reinforcing the importance of maintaining confidentiality.

Cultural Sensitivity

Patients bring diverse cultural, spiritual, and personal values into healthcare settings, and respecting these differences is crucial for delivering patient-centered care. Nurses advocate for cultural sensitivity by seeking to understand and honor patients' preferences, even when they differ from standard medical practices. This might include arranging for dietary accommodations, involving spiritual advisors in care discussions, or respecting a patient's decision to decline certain treatments due to religious beliefs. For instance, a nurse may advocate for the inclusion of a traditional healer as part of a patient's care team, recognizing its importance to the patient's well-being. By promoting cultural sensitivity, nurses create an environment where all patients feel respected and valued.

1.2.2 Examples of Advocacy in Action

Example 1: Intervening When a Patient is Pressured into a Procedure Without Fully Understanding the Risks

Mrs. Johnson, a 72-year-old patient, is advised by her physician to undergo an invasive surgical procedure to address her chronic pain. During the discussion, she appears hesitant and expresses confusion about the risks and benefits of the surgery. However, the physician continues to emphasize the urgency of the procedure, leaving her feeling pressured to consent.

The nurse, noticing Mrs. Johnson's discomfort, steps in to provide additional clarity. They explain the procedure in simpler terms, outline possible alternatives, and give Mrs. Johnson the time she needs to ask questions and consider her options. By ensuring that she fully understands the situation and feels empowered to make an informed decision, the nurse protects Mrs. Johnson's right to autonomy and prevents her from agreeing to a procedure under duress.

Example 2: Advocating for Equitable Treatment of a Patient Facing Systemic Barriers

Mr. Ahmed, a 45-year-old immigrant with limited English proficiency, arrives at the emergency department with severe chest pain. Due to a language barrier, the initial medical team struggles to gather a full medical history and quickly proceeds with standard treatment protocols. The nurse recognizes that Mr. Ahmed may not fully understand the care being provided and that cultural factors could influence his treatment preferences.

The nurse advocates for the use of an interpreter to ensure clear communication and discovers that Mr. Ahmed has a history of allergic reactions to specific medications commonly used for his condition. By addressing this barrier and personalizing his care, the nurse not only prevents potential complications but also ensures that Mr. Ahmed receives treatment that aligns with his needs and circumstances.

Example 3: Supporting a Patient's Right to Refuse Care Due to Cultural or Personal Beliefs

Ms. Lopez, a 33-year-old patient, declines a blood transfusion due to her religious beliefs, despite her physician's recommendation that it is necessary to manage her condition. While the care team is concerned about the risks of refusing the treatment, the nurse steps forward to advocate for Ms. Lopez's rights.

The nurse arranges a meeting with the patient, her family, and the healthcare team to explore alternative treatments that align with her values. This might include the use of bloodless medicine techniques or other non-invasive options. By respecting Ms. Lopez's decision and facilitating a solution that honors her beliefs, the nurse ensures that her care remains both effective and aligned with her personal values.

1.2.3 Nurse's Ethical Responsibilities in Advocacy

Nurses are bound by ethical principles that guide their advocacy efforts and ensure patients receive equitable, respectful, and compassionate care. Advocacy is not only a professional duty but also an ethical commitment to prioritizing the well-being and rights of those they serve.

The principles of autonomy, beneficence, and justice are central to nursing advocacy:

- **Autonomy:** Nurses support patients' right to make decisions about their own care, even when those decisions differ from medical recommendations. By providing information, respecting choices, and ensuring those choices are honored, nurses empower patients to maintain control over their healthcare. For instance, a nurse who upholds autonomy will respect a patient's informed decision to refuse life-sustaining treatment.
- **Beneficence:** Acting in the patient's best interests is a key tenet of nursing practice. Advocacy involves ensuring that all interventions aim to benefit the patient, minimize harm, and align with their values and goals. For example, advocating for pain management in a palliative care setting ensures the patient's comfort and dignity.
- **Justice:** Advocacy includes promoting fairness and equity in care delivery. Nurses work to ensure that patients, regardless of background, receive the resources and treatments they need. This principle is particularly important when addressing disparities in healthcare access or systemic inequalities.

While advocating for patients, nurses must also navigate the constraints of organizational policies, available resources, and institutional priorities. Balancing these demands requires skill and discretion:

- Nurses often mediate between patients and healthcare administrators, advocating for necessary treatments or accommodations while recognizing budgetary or staffing limitations.
- For example, if a patient requires a costly medication not covered by insurance, a nurse might collaborate with social workers to identify alternative funding sources or programs that provide the treatment at reduced costs. By balancing patient advocacy with organizational realities, nurses ensure they remain effective in their role while promoting equitable care.

Ethical dilemmas frequently arise when patient preferences conflict with clinical recommendations or family wishes. Nurses are uniquely positioned to navigate these challenges while maintaining a patient-centered approach:

- **Conflicts Between Patient Preferences and Clinical Recommendations:** A patient may decline a recommended treatment due to personal or cultural beliefs, even when the care team views the intervention as essential. Nurses address this by facilitating open communication, seeking to understand the patient's perspective, and exploring alternative treatments that align with the patient's values.

- **Conflicts Among Family Members or the Care Team:** Disagreements between family members or between the care team and a patient's surrogate decision-maker can create ethical tensions. Nurses advocate for the patient's documented or expressed wishes, ensuring their autonomy is respected. For example, a nurse might mediate discussions when family members disagree on the use of life-sustaining interventions for an incapacitated patient.

In these scenarios, nurses may also consult institutional ethics committees or legal advisors to ensure their advocacy aligns with professional standards and organizational guidelines.

1.3 Empowering Patients to Speak for Themselves

Empowering patients to take an active role in their healthcare fosters better outcomes, improved satisfaction, and stronger patient-provider relationships. When patients are encouraged to speak for themselves, they can make informed decisions, express their preferences, and contribute to the development of care plans that align with their values and goals.

Active participation not only enhances autonomy but also increases a patient's understanding of their condition and treatment options. This understanding often reduces anxiety and builds trust in the care process. For example, a patient who feels confident asking questions about their diagnosis is more likely to adhere to prescribed treatments and recognize warning signs that require medical attention.

Moreover, when patients advocate for themselves, they become partners in their care rather than passive recipients. This collaborative dynamic leads to a more personalized approach to treatment, ensuring that care addresses both medical and personal needs.

Strategies to Foster Confidence in Self-Advocacy

1. **Educating Patients About Their Rights and Options**

   Providing patients with clear, accessible information about their rights and treatment choices is foundational for self-advocacy. Nurses can explain medical terms in plain language, guide patients through available resources, and encourage them to ask questions. For instance, offering a patient-friendly guide to their diagnosis or a step-by-step explanation of a procedure helps them feel more informed and prepared to engage in their care.

2. **Encouraging Open Communication**

   Nurses can create a safe environment where patients feel comfortable expressing their thoughts, concerns, and preferences. Using active listening techniques, such as making eye contact, paraphrasing, and validating feelings, reassures patients that their voice matters. For example, a nurse might say, "It's important that we hear your thoughts on this treatment plan—what concerns or questions do you have?"

3. **Building Patient Confidence Through Positive Reinforcement**

   Encouraging and affirming patients' decisions and actions reinforces their confidence in self-advocacy. Simple statements like, "That's a great question to ask the doctor," or, "I'm glad you brought that up," validate their efforts and show that their input is valued.

4. **Providing Tools for Effective Communication**

   Equipping patients with practical tools, such as a list of questions to ask during appointments or a journal to track symptoms, empowers them to engage more effectively in their care. For example, a nurse could recommend that a patient bring a trusted family member to appointments or prepare notes about concerns to discuss with their provider.

5. **Respecting Cultural and Personal Beliefs**

   Empowerment begins with recognizing and respecting a patient's individual values, beliefs, and cultural background. By demonstrating sensitivity and a willingness to adapt care approaches, nurses foster trust and encourage patients to advocate for their unique needs. For example, acknowledging a patient's preference for holistic treatments and discussing how they can integrate those preferences into their care plan shows respect for their voice.

6. **Encouraging Peer Support and Shared Experiences**

   Connecting patients with support groups or others who have faced similar challenges can inspire confidence and provide valuable insights. Hearing stories of self-advocacy and success from peers reinforces the idea that speaking up can lead to better outcomes.

1.4 Delegating Responsibilities in Patient Care

Delegation is an essential skill in nursing practice, allowing for efficient care delivery by leveraging the skills and strengths of the healthcare team. Effective delegation ensures that tasks are performed safely and competently while allowing nurses to focus on their higher-level responsibilities. The following principles and best practices guide the delegation process:

1.4.1 Accountability and Responsibility

When delegating tasks in patient care, nurses must remember that while the execution of a specific task can be assigned to another team member, the ultimate accountability for the outcome remains with the nurse. Delegation is not simply about assigning work; it is about ensuring that the task is performed correctly, safely, and in alignment with established standards of care. This principle underscores the importance of oversight, as any errors or omissions in the delegated task can directly impact patient outcomes and reflect on the nurse's professional responsibilities.

For example, consider a nurse delegating the task of checking a patient's vital signs to a nursing assistant. While the assistant is responsible for performing the task, the nurse must ensure that the readings are accurately recorded and evaluated. If a critical change in the patient's blood pressure or heart rate is noted, the nurse is responsible for interpreting this information and taking appropriate action, such as notifying the physician or adjusting the care plan. Failure to monitor or follow up on the delegated task could result in missed opportunities to address emerging health concerns, potentially jeopardizing patient safety.

Moreover, accountability extends to confirming that the person assigned to the task has the necessary skills, knowledge, and training to perform it competently. Delegating without verifying the delegate's competency can lead to mistakes or delays in care. For instance, asking an untrained staff member to monitor a complex piece of equipment could result in equipment misuse and adverse patient outcomes.

Nurses must also maintain clear communication with the individual carrying out the task, offering support and guidance as needed. This collaborative approach ensures that tasks are completed accurately and fosters a sense of trust and mutual respect within the healthcare team. By retaining accountability and actively overseeing the delegated tasks, nurses fulfill their ethical and professional obligation to deliver high-quality, patient-centered care while leveraging the strengths of their team effectively.

1.4.2 Clarity of Communication

Effective delegation begins with clear and precise communication. Nurses must provide detailed instructions that outline the task, its expected outcomes, and the timeframe within which it needs to be completed. Clear communication minimizes misunderstandings and ensures that the delegate has a comprehensive understanding of what is expected, reducing the risk of errors and promoting patient safety.

When delegating, it is essential for the nurse to clearly articulate the steps involved in the task and any specific considerations that must be taken into account. For example, if delegating a task such as checking blood glucose levels, the nurse should specify not only how and when the task should be performed but also what to do with the results, such as reporting abnormal readings immediately or documenting them in a specific format. These instructions ensure that the delegate knows exactly what to do and how their work contributes to the overall care plan.

It is equally important to verify that the delegate fully understands their role and the scope of practice within which they are expected to operate. For instance, a nursing assistant may be tasked with measuring a patient's vital signs, but the interpretation of those readings and any clinical decisions based on them remain the responsibility of the nurse. Ensuring that the delegate understands these boundaries prevents them from inadvertently overstepping their responsibilities.

One of the most effective ways to confirm comprehension is to use open-ended questions. Instead of simply asking, "Do you understand?"—which may lead to a yes or no response—nurses can encourage the delegate to explain their approach to the task. A question like, "Can you explain how you'll approach this task?" allows the nurse to gauge the delegate's understanding and address any gaps in knowledge before the task begins. This technique fosters a collaborative environment, promotes learning, and instills confidence in the delegate.

1.4.3 Prioritization of Patient Safety

When delegating tasks, the foremost priority must always be patient safety. This requires careful consideration of the skills, training, and expertise of the individual to whom a task is being assigned. Delegation is not a one-size-fits-all process; it involves matching the complexity of the task to the capabilities of the team member. By doing so, nurses ensure that care is delivered competently and without compromising the well-being of the patient.

Tasks that require specialized knowledge, such as complex wound care or administering medications, should be assigned to licensed professionals who possess the necessary clinical training to handle these responsibilities. For instance, a registered nurse might delegate wound dressing changes to a licensed practical nurse (LPN) who has experience in managing wound care. Assigning this task to an unlicensed assistant who lacks the required knowledge could result in improper techniques, increased risk of infection, or delayed healing—all of which directly jeopardize patient safety.

Conversely, non-clinical or routine tasks that do not require advanced training can be effectively delegated to support staff. Activities such as restocking supplies, transporting patients, or assisting with hygiene needs are essential to maintaining efficient operations but do not pose a direct risk to patient health if performed by team members with less clinical expertise. For example, a nursing assistant may be tasked with ensuring that a patient room is stocked with the necessary equipment, freeing the nurse to focus on more complex care needs.

Delegation decisions must also account for the context and urgency of the situation. In high-stakes scenarios, such as responding to a sudden change in a patient's condition, tasks requiring immediate clinical judgment should remain with the nurse or other licensed professionals. This ensures that critical interventions are carried out by those with the expertise to assess and act on the situation appropriately.

1.4.4 Adherence to Legal and Ethical Standards

Delegation in nursing is not only a practical decision but also one deeply rooted in legal and ethical considerations. Nurses must navigate a complex framework of state laws, facility policies, and professional ethical guidelines to ensure that tasks are delegated appropriately and responsibly. Adhering to these standards is essential to maintaining the integrity of patient care and protecting both patients and healthcare professionals from potential harm.

State laws and regulations play a significant role in defining the scope of practice for various healthcare team members. These laws outline the specific duties that licensed professionals, nursing assistants, and other support staff are legally permitted to perform. For example, while a licensed practical nurse (LPN) may administer certain medications, a nursing assistant is restricted from doing so under most state laws. Nurses must be thoroughly familiar with these regulations to ensure that delegation remains within legal boundaries and does not place team members in situations that exceed their competencies.

Facility policies further refine the delegation process by setting specific guidelines tailored to the organization's operations, patient population, and resources. These policies often include protocols for training, supervision, and reporting, ensuring that tasks are performed consistently and safely. For instance, a hospital policy may require nurses to directly observe certain high-risk procedures when delegated, providing an additional layer of oversight and accountability.

Ethical guidelines, such as those outlined by the American Nurses Association (ANA), emphasize the nurse's responsibility to prioritize patient safety, autonomy, and dignity during the delegation process. Delegation should always align with the principles of beneficence (acting in the patient's best interest), non-maleficence (avoiding harm), and justice (ensuring equitable care). For example, it would be ethically inappropriate to delegate a complex task to an inexperienced staff member simply to save time or reduce the workload.

1.4.5 Supervision and Feedback

Delegation is not complete once a task is assigned; it requires ongoing supervision to ensure tasks are carried out effectively, safely, and according to established standards. Nurses play a key role in monitoring the performance of delegated responsibilities, remaining available to address questions, offer clarification, or provide real-time guidance as needed. This continuous oversight ensures that patient care remains of the highest quality and helps prevent errors or misunderstandings. For example, a nurse who delegates blood pressure monitoring should periodically review the readings to confirm accuracy and address any irregularities promptly.

Providing constructive feedback is an essential component of successful delegation. Feedback should be specific, timely, and delivered in a supportive manner, helping team members understand what was done well and where improvement is needed. For instance, a nurse might commend a nursing assistant for handling a task with professionalism, while also offering suggestions to refine their technique for even better results. Positive reinforcement encourages confidence and motivation, while corrective feedback, when framed constructively, fosters learning and professional development.

1.4.6 Assigning Tasks Effectively Based on Team Member Competencies

To delegate responsibilities effectively, nurses must assess team members' competencies, strengths, and limitations. This involves understanding each individual's scope of practice, level of training, and experience, as well as the specific requirements of the task at hand.

1. **Assessing Competencies:** Begin by evaluating the delegate's qualifications, skills, and experience. For instance, a nursing assistant may be proficient in assisting with activities of daily living (ADLs) but may require supervision for new or unfamiliar procedures. Matching tasks to capabilities minimizes errors and builds team confidence.
2. **Providing Clear Instructions:** Specify the task in detail, including any critical steps, expected outcomes, and reporting requirements. For example, if assigning medication administration

to a licensed practical nurse (LPN), clarify the specific medications, dosages, and any monitoring responsibilities.

3. **Considering Workloads:** Take into account the current workload and availability of team members. Delegating a task to an overburdened staff member may result in delays or errors. For example, distributing tasks evenly among available staff ensures that responsibilities are manageable and efficiently completed.
4. **Encouraging Collaboration:** Foster an environment where team members feel comfortable asking questions or seeking clarification. This collaboration ensures that tasks are performed correctly and reinforces trust among the team. For instance, an inexperienced team member may need reassurance and support while learning a new skill under supervision.
5. **Monitoring and Supporting Task Completion:** Delegation requires ongoing supervision to ensure tasks are carried out as intended. For example, a nurse who delegates blood pressure monitoring should periodically check the recorded results and address any abnormalities promptly. Offering feedback, such as praising accurate work or suggesting improvements, strengthens team performance and accountability.

1.5 Collaborating with Healthcare Teams

As frontline caregivers, LPNs act as a critical link, facilitating communication and coordination among various healthcare professionals while keeping the patient at the center of care. Their position allows them to bridge gaps, ensuring that care plans are effectively implemented and that patient needs are promptly addressed.

One of the key functions of LPNs in interdisciplinary teamwork is to serve as a communication conduit. LPNs are often the team members who spend the most time with patients, providing hands-on care and observing changes in their condition. Through detailed reporting and documentation, they ensure that other team members, such as registered nurses (RNs), physicians, and therapists, are kept informed about the patient's status. For example, if a patient recovering from surgery develops unexpected swelling, the LPN can promptly communicate this finding to the appropriate team member, allowing for timely intervention.

LPNs also play an essential role in implementing care plans that have been developed by the healthcare team. While other professionals, such as physicians or RNs, may design treatment strategies, LPNs are responsible for carrying out specific components of these plans, such as administering medications, assisting with wound care, or providing daily support for activities of living. For instance, when a physical therapist prescribes mobility exercises for a patient, the LPN may assist the patient with performing these exercises, ensuring that the prescribed therapy is executed consistently and safely.

In addition to executing care plans, LPNs contribute to the collaborative process by monitoring patient progress and reporting any concerns or deviations. Their observations and insights are invaluable during team discussions, as they provide firsthand information about the patient's responses to treatment. For example, if a patient undergoing therapy for a swallowing disorder struggles with prescribed exercises, the LPN can inform the speech therapist, enabling adjustments to the care plan.

1.5.1 Contributions of Healthcare Team Members

In an interdisciplinary healthcare setting, various team members contribute their unique expertise to create a holistic approach to patient care. Each professional brings specialized knowledge and skills that complement nursing care, addressing a wide range of patient needs. This collaborative effort ensures comprehensive treatment plans that improve patient outcomes and quality of life.

Occupational therapists, physical therapists, and speech therapists are key members of the healthcare team, each focusing on specific areas of patient recovery and well-being. Occupational therapists primarily work to enhance a patient's ability to perform daily activities, such as dressing, eating, or managing household tasks. Their interventions are particularly valuable for patients recovering from strokes, injuries, or surgeries that limit their independence. For instance, an occupational therapist may recommend adaptive tools or techniques to help a patient with limited hand mobility regain the ability to eat independently. In such scenarios, LPNs assist by encouraging patients to use these tools during meals, reinforcing the therapist's strategies in daily practice.

Physical therapists focus on restoring movement, strength, and mobility. They play a critical role in helping patients recover from musculoskeletal injuries, surgeries, or neurological conditions. For example, a physical therapist might design an exercise regimen to improve a patient's ability to walk after a hip replacement. The LPN supports this plan by assisting the patient with mobility exercises, ensuring safety during ambulation, and monitoring for signs of discomfort or fatigue. This partnership allows for consistent application of the therapy and helps track the patient's progress.

Speech therapists, also known as speech-language pathologists, address communication and swallowing disorders. Their expertise is crucial for patients with conditions like dysphagia, aphasia, or cognitive impairments. For instance, a speech therapist may work with a patient who has difficulty swallowing to develop techniques for safer eating, such as adjusting food texture or teaching specific swallowing strategies. The LPN complements this care by monitoring the patient's nutritional intake, ensuring compliance with dietary modifications, and providing hands-on assistance during meals. If the patient struggles with a prescribed strategy, the LPN can communicate this to the speech therapist, facilitating timely adjustments to the care plan.

The collaboration between these specialists and LPNs is essential in addressing complex patient needs. Each team member's contribution is interconnected, with LPNs often implementing and reinforcing the specialized care plans developed by therapists. For example, in the case of a stroke patient with mobility challenges and dysphagia, the physical therapist may focus on improving movement, the speech therapist on swallowing safety, and the LPN on integrating both aspects into daily routines, such as guiding the patient to safely walk to the dining area and assisting with a modified meal.

1.5.2 Emphasizing Communication in Teamwork

Effective communication is the foundation of successful teamwork in healthcare, ensuring that all team members are aligned in their roles and responsibilities. Clear and concise communication minimizes misunderstandings, prevents errors, and fosters a safe, collaborative environment where patient care remains the top priority. For Licensed Practical Nurses (LPNs), their position as a critical link between the healthcare team, patients, and families makes their communication skills essential to delivering high-quality care.

In interdisciplinary teams, clarity in communication ensures that everyone understands their specific responsibilities within the care plan. For instance, an LPN collaborating with a physical therapist and a registered nurse (RN) to improve a patient's mobility must clearly understand and convey the therapist's prescribed exercises. Miscommunication in this scenario—such as incorrectly instructing the patient—could lead to errors that delay progress or even cause harm. By ensuring that the instructions are accurately relayed and consistently followed, the LPN contributes to the patient's recovery and reinforces the team's collective efforts.

Communication is equally important when it comes to patient and family involvement. LPNs often serve as the primary point of contact for patients and their loved ones, translating medical jargon into clear, understandable terms. For example, after a team meeting where changes to a patient's care plan are discussed, the LPN might update the family, explaining new medication routines or therapy schedules. This ensures that patients and families are fully informed, reducing anxiety and fostering trust in the care team.

Moreover, effective communication helps to address and prevent potential errors. LPNs are trained to recognize and report discrepancies in care, such as conflicting orders or unexpected changes in a patient's condition. For instance, if a patient's medication dosage appears to differ from the original prescription, the LPN can promptly communicate this to the prescribing physician or pharmacist, preventing a possible error. Similarly, when a patient reports new symptoms, the LPN ensures that this information reaches the appropriate team member quickly, enabling timely interventions.

An example of the LPN's role in facilitating communication can be seen in their efforts to align care plans. If a patient with a complex medical condition requires input from multiple specialists, such as a cardiologist and a dietitian, the LPN might relay updates from one provider to another, ensuring that care decisions are coordinated and consistent. This level of communication is crucial in preventing conflicting advice or overlapping interventions that could confuse the patient or compromise care.

Example 1: Coordinating Patient Education After a Team Meeting

A 65-year-old patient with newly diagnosed diabetes meets with an interdisciplinary team that includes an endocrinologist, a dietitian, and a pharmacist. During the meeting, the team agrees on a care plan that includes blood sugar monitoring, insulin administration, and dietary adjustments. After the meeting, the LPN takes the lead in relaying these updates to the patient and their family.

The LPN explains how to use the blood glucose monitor, demonstrates the correct insulin injection technique, and reinforces the dietitian's recommendations for meal planning. Recognizing that the patient appears overwhelmed, the LPN also provides written instructions and answers questions to ensure clarity. By serving as the bridge between the healthcare team and the patient, the LPN ensures that the patient fully understands the care plan, reducing anxiety and enhancing adherence to the prescribed regimen.

Example 2: Preventing Medication Errors Through Communication

In a busy hospital setting, a patient recovering from surgery reports increased nausea after receiving pain medication. The LPN notices that the prescribed dosage appears higher than standard for the patient's weight and age. Recognizing the potential for a medication error, the LPN immediately communicates the concern to the RN and physician.

After a review of the medication order, the physician confirms that the dosage was indeed incorrect and adjusts it accordingly. The LPN then updates the patient, explaining the change and addressing their concerns about side effects. By identifying and reporting the discrepancy quickly, the LPN prevents further discomfort for the patient and ensures their safety, demonstrating the critical role of clear and proactive communication in preventing errors.

1.6 Safeguarding Patient Privacy and Information

Patient confidentiality is a foundational principle of healthcare ethics, deeply rooted in the concept of respect for patient autonomy. Autonomy grants individuals the right to make decisions about their own lives, including how their personal health information is used and shared. This principle fosters trust between patients and healthcare providers, creating a safe environment where patients feel comfortable sharing sensitive details essential for their care. Patients have the right to control who accesses their personal health information (PHI) and for what purposes. It is the responsibility of healthcare providers, including Licensed Practical Nurses (LPNs), to ensure that any disclosure of this information is strictly limited to individuals directly involved in the patient's care or for legitimate healthcare operations, such as treatment, payment, or administrative purposes. For example, sharing a patient's medical history with a physical therapist participating in their rehabilitation is an appropriate use of PHI, but discussing the same information with an unrelated colleague or friend constitutes a breach of confidentiality.

The Health Insurance Portability and Accountability Act (HIPAA) serves as the legal framework for safeguarding PHI, setting strict guidelines for its storage, transmission, and disposal. These regulations apply to all forms of PHI, whether paper records, electronic data, or verbal communication. HIPAA mandates secure storage of physical records in locked cabinets or restricted-access areas and requires electronic information to be protected by encryption and password security. Transmission of PHI must occur through secure channels, such as encrypted email systems, to prevent unauthorized access. Similarly, disposal methods, such as shredding paper documents or securely deleting electronic files, must ensure that sensitive information cannot be reconstructed.

LPNs play a critical role in adhering to these regulations by following best practices, such as logging out of shared workstations, regularly updating passwords, and avoiding discussions about patients in public areas where unauthorized individuals could overhear. For example, an LPN should refrain from discussing a patient's condition in a busy hallway or an elevator, even in casual conversation with a colleague. Vigilance in these seemingly minor interactions is crucial to preventing breaches of confidentiality.

Failure to maintain patient confidentiality can lead to significant legal, professional, and personal consequences. For LPNs, a breach of confidentiality could result in disciplinary action, including suspension or loss of licensure. For healthcare organizations, violations may lead to substantial financial penalties, reputational damage, and loss of patient trust. Patients who experience a breach of privacy may face emotional distress and the potential misuse of their information. For instance, a cybersecurity breach that exposes patient data not only incurs financial penalties under HIPAA but also erodes the confidence patients have in the institution's ability to protect their most sensitive information.

Upholding confidentiality extends beyond meeting regulatory requirements; it reflects the respect and professionalism inherent in quality healthcare. Patients who trust that their information is secure are more likely to share critical health details, allowing providers to make accurate diagnoses and deliver effective care. LPNs, as frontline caregivers, are essential to preserving this trust. By diligently protecting PHI, maintaining awareness of confidentiality protocols, and addressing potential breaches proactively, LPNs ensure that patient privacy is safeguarded, reinforcing the integrity and ethical foundation of the healthcare system.

1.6.1 Scenarios Illustrating the Protection of Personal Health Information

Scenario 1: Avoiding Unauthorized Disclosure

An LPN working in a hospital overhears two colleagues discussing a patient's recent diagnosis in the elevator. Recognizing that this violates the patient's privacy, the LPN immediately intervenes, reminding the colleagues of the importance of maintaining confidentiality and avoiding discussions in public areas. Later, the LPN reports the incident to a supervisor to ensure proper action is taken. This scenario highlights the proactive role LPNs play in protecting patient privacy and educating others about ethical practices.

Scenario 2: Securely Managing Patient Records

While preparing discharge paperwork, an LPN accidentally prints a patient's medical records and leaves them on a shared printer. Realizing the mistake, the LPN quickly retrieves the documents, confirms that no one else has accessed them, and securely shreds unnecessary copies. The LPN also reflects on the incident and adjusts their workflow to double-check print jobs in the future, ensuring sensitive information remains secure. This example illustrates the importance of vigilance and immediate corrective actions in safeguarding patient data.

Scenario 3: Ensuring Privacy During Discussions

An LPN is discussing a patient's treatment plan with a family member. When the conversation begins in the patient's semi-private room, the patient expresses discomfort with others overhearing the details. The LPN promptly offers to continue the discussion in a private setting, ensuring the patient feels secure and respected. By accommodating the patient's preference for confidentiality, the LPN reinforces trust and adheres to ethical standards.

1.7 Ensuring Patient Comfort and Privacy

Maintaining patient dignity requires an empathetic and proactive approach. Simple yet impactful measures, such as knocking before entering a patient's room, addressing patients by their preferred names, and ensuring proper draping during examinations, demonstrate respect for personal boundaries. These actions convey to patients that their autonomy and sense of self are valued, even in vulnerable situations. For instance, when assisting a patient with personal hygiene, an LPN can provide privacy by closing curtains or doors and explaining each step of the process beforehand to ensure the patient feels secure and informed. These practices not only preserve dignity but also enhance the patient's sense of control over their care.

Cultural considerations play a vital role in maintaining patient comfort and privacy, as diverse backgrounds influence individual expectations about personal space, modesty, and communication styles. Licensed Practical Nurses (LPNs) must approach these cultural differences with sensitivity and adaptability, ensuring that care is delivered in a manner that respects the patient's values and beliefs. By understanding and honoring these differences, nurses foster trust, reduce anxiety, and create an inclusive and respectful environment.

For many patients, modesty is a deeply ingrained cultural or religious value, particularly during intimate procedures. For instance, patients from Muslim, Orthodox Jewish, or Hindu backgrounds may prefer same-gender caregivers for activities such as bathing, dressing, or physical examinations. This preference often stems from religious teachings or cultural norms emphasizing modesty. In such cases, the LPN should make every effort to accommodate these requests by coordinating with the care team to assign same-gender staff. If a same-gender caregiver is unavailable, the LPN can take steps to ensure privacy by using extra draping, allowing the patient to wear additional clothing when appropriate, and seeking consent for each step of the procedure. These adjustments demonstrate respect for the patient's beliefs and help build a trusting relationship.

Personal space is another cultural aspect that can vary significantly. For example, patients from Latin American or Mediterranean cultures may be more comfortable with closer physical proximity and touch during interactions, seeing it as a sign of warmth and compassion. Conversely, patients from East Asian or Northern European cultures may value a greater sense of personal space and may feel uncomfortable with unnecessary physical contact. LPNs should be observant of these preferences and adjust their approach accordingly. For instance, asking permission before initiating physical touch, such as during a blood pressure check, can help establish comfort and respect for those who prefer a larger personal boundary.

Communication styles also differ widely across cultures, and LPNs must recognize and adapt to these variations. Nonverbal cues such as eye contact, gestures, and tone of voice often hold cultural significance. For example, in some Indigenous or Asian cultures, avoiding direct eye contact may be a sign of respect, whereas in Western cultures, it is often interpreted as a lack of confidence or engagement. An LPN working with a patient who avoids eye contact should avoid assuming disinterest and instead focus on other cues, such as the patient's verbal responses or body language, to assess their comfort and understanding.

Language barriers can also present challenges to effective communication and privacy. For patients with limited proficiency in the primary language of the care setting, the use of professional interpreters or translated materials is essential. LPNs should avoid relying on family members to translate sensitive information, as this can compromise both accuracy and the patient's comfort in sharing private details. For example, a patient may be hesitant to discuss symptoms related to reproductive health if their child or spouse is acting as the interpreter. Using a trained interpreter ensures confidentiality and promotes a clearer understanding of the patient's needs.

Additionally, cultural views on decision-making can influence patient preferences for privacy and autonomy. In some cultures, healthcare decisions are viewed as a collective family responsibility rather than an individual choice. For example, patients from Middle Eastern or East Asian cultures may defer decision-making to a family elder or involve multiple family members in discussions about treatment. LPNs should respect these practices by creating an environment that allows for family involvement, while also ensuring that the patient's voice remains central to the discussion.

In addition to cultural awareness, LPNs must be attuned to individual patient preferences and emotional well-being. Respecting these preferences might involve adjusting care routines to align with the patient's daily habits or involving family members in decision-making when appropriate. For example, a patient recovering from surgery may feel more comfortable if their family member is present during physical therapy sessions. The nurse's role in facilitating such accommodations demonstrates a patient-centered approach that prioritizes emotional comfort alongside medical needs.

The nurse-patient relationship is built on trust, and privacy is a key component of that trust. Protecting a patient's privacy extends beyond safeguarding health information to include their physical and emotional space. For example, during a dressing change or other procedures, an LPN should ensure that only the necessary body part is exposed and that the patient is informed about what is being done at each step. This approach minimizes feelings of vulnerability and promotes a sense of safety.

Creating a respectful environment also involves advocating for patients who may not feel comfortable expressing their needs. LPNs should encourage open communication by asking patients about their preferences and addressing concerns in a nonjudgmental manner. For instance, if a patient hesitates to discuss a sensitive issue, the nurse can create a supportive atmosphere by expressing empathy and ensuring the conversation remains confidential. This proactive approach empowers patients to voice their concerns and participate actively in their care.

1.8 Continuity of Care After Discharge

Continuity of care after discharge is a vital component of effective nursing practice, ensuring that patients transition safely from the healthcare facility to their home or another care setting. It reduces the risk of complications, improves recovery outcomes, and prevents hospital readmissions. For LPNs, understanding how to provide seamless post-discharge support is critical. This involves clear communication with patients and their families, practical problem-solving, and a focus on follow-up care to address individual needs.

Follow-up care ensures that the progress made during hospitalization continues post-discharge. For example, a patient recovering from pneumonia may be prescribed antibiotics, instructed to monitor their breathing, and scheduled for a follow-up appointment with their primary care provider. If the patient fails to adhere to their medication schedule or skips the appointment due to lack of understanding or resources, they risk complications such as recurring infections or worsening symptoms.

Consider a scenario where an elderly patient with diabetes is discharged after being treated for a diabetic wound. Before discharge, the care team, including the LPN, creates a plan that includes dressing changes, blood sugar monitoring, and a follow-up with a wound care specialist. The LPN explains the importance of keeping the wound clean and demonstrates proper dressing techniques. If the patient struggles to manage the wound care independently, follow-up efforts such as phone calls or referrals to home health services ensure that the patient's needs are met and complications are minimized.

1.8.1 Effective Communication with Patients and Families

Clear communication is essential for helping patients understand and follow their discharge plans. LPNs must take the time to explain the care plan in detail, ensuring that patients and their caregivers have a clear understanding of what is required at home. For instance, a patient discharged after surgery might need to manage pain, monitor for signs of infection, and attend physical therapy. The LPN should explain the purpose of each component of the plan, provide written instructions, and encourage the patient to ask questions.

For example, a patient prescribed anticoagulants after knee surgery may not understand the importance of avoiding certain over-the-counter medications that can increase the risk of bleeding. The LPN should educate the patient about these risks and provide a list of safe alternatives. Additionally, if a patient expresses concerns about remembering their medication schedule, the LPN might suggest using a pill organizer or setting reminders on their phone.

Post-discharge follow-up communication is equally important. A follow-up phone call within 48 hours provides an opportunity to address questions and ensure the patient is adhering to the care plan. For example, during a follow-up call, an LPN might learn that a patient recovering from a cardiac event has been experiencing fatigue during physical therapy. The LPN can relay this information to the healthcare team, leading to adjustments in the therapy plan and preventing further strain on the patient.

1.8.2 Identifying and Overcoming Barriers

LPNs play a critical role in identifying barriers that may hinder continuity of care. Social determinants of health, such as lack of transportation, financial constraints, or limited access to healthcare resources, can create significant challenges. For example, a patient discharged with a prescription for expensive medications may struggle to afford them. The LPN can collaborate with social workers or case managers to identify low-cost alternatives, such as generic medications or pharmaceutical assistance programs.

Another common barrier is difficulty accessing follow-up care. For instance, a patient without transportation may miss a critical follow-up appointment with a specialist. In this case, the LPN can connect the patient with community resources that provide transportation services or explore telehealth options if appropriate.

Case Example: Preventing Readmission After a Heart Failure Diagnosis

Consider a patient discharged with a diagnosis of heart failure. The discharge plan includes a low-sodium diet, daily weight monitoring, medication adherence, and a follow-up with a cardiologist. The LPN educates the patient about recognizing early signs of worsening heart failure, such as sudden weight gain or shortness of breath.

Two days post-discharge, the LPN conducts a follow-up call and learns that the patient has gained three pounds in 24 hours but has not yet started their prescribed diuretic due to confusion about the instructions. The LPN clarifies the medication schedule, emphasizes the importance of taking the diuretic as prescribed, and advises the patient to contact their cardiologist immediately. This intervention prevents the patient's condition from escalating, reducing the risk of readmission.

1.9 Communicating Effectively During Handoffs

The handoff process involves transferring responsibility for a patient's care from one healthcare provider to another, typically during shift changes, transfers between units, or when a patient transitions to a new level of care. LPNs play a pivotal role in this process, as accurate and thorough handoffs can prevent errors, reduce misunderstandings, and maintain patient safety.

Accurate shift reporting is essential to provide the incoming nurse with a comprehensive understanding of the patient's current condition, recent changes, ongoing interventions, and anticipated needs. For example, if a patient is recovering from surgery, the LPN handing off care must report on their pain levels, mobility status, medication administration, and any complications such as nausea or difficulty urinating. A vague or incomplete report could lead to delays in addressing critical needs or duplicate efforts, potentially compromising the patient's safety and care quality.

Handoffs also serve as an opportunity to communicate observations that may not be immediately documented in the patient's chart but are crucial for continuity of care. For instance, an LPN might note that a patient with dementia is more agitated during evening hours or that a patient recovering from a stroke requires encouragement during physical therapy. Sharing these details helps the incoming nurse anticipate challenges and tailor their approach to the patient's needs.

To enhance the effectiveness of handoffs, structured communication tools like SBAR (Situation, Background, Assessment, Recommendation) have become widely adopted. SBAR provides a standardized framework that ensures all critical information is conveyed systematically and concisely, reducing the likelihood of important details being overlooked.

- **Situation:** Clearly describe the immediate issue or reason for the handoff. For example, "The patient is a 75-year-old male admitted with pneumonia who is experiencing shortness of breath despite oxygen therapy at 3L/min."
- **Background:** Provide relevant context, such as medical history or recent changes. "The patient has a history of COPD and was started on antibiotics and bronchodilators yesterday. His oxygen saturation has been stable at 92% until this afternoon."
- **Assessment:** Share observations or clinical findings. "This evening, his oxygen saturation dropped to 88%, and he reports increased fatigue and difficulty breathing."
- **Recommendation:** Suggest next steps or actions for the incoming nurse. "I recommend monitoring his oxygen levels closely and considering a consult with respiratory therapy if his condition doesn't improve."

Using SBAR ensures that all pertinent information is included while keeping the communication focused and organized. It also promotes clarity by encouraging concise, objective descriptions of the patient's condition and care plan.

Another example of effective handoff communication is during a unit transfer. Suppose a patient is being transferred from a surgical unit to a rehabilitation facility. The LPN responsible for the handoff should use a structured approach to convey critical information, such as the patient's surgical procedure, current medications, mobility limitations, wound care instructions, and upcoming follow-up appointments. In this case, SBAR or a facility-specific transfer checklist can help ensure no essential details are missed.

Clear and effective communication during handoffs is not just about relaying facts but also about verifying understanding. The incoming nurse should have the opportunity to ask questions or clarify details as needed. For instance, if an incoming nurse is unsure about the timing of a patient's last dose of pain medication, the LPN providing the handoff can review the chart together to ensure accuracy.

Miscommunication during handoffs is one of the leading causes of medical errors, making this process a critical focus for quality improvement in healthcare settings. By emphasizing accuracy, adopting structured communication tools like SBAR, and fostering a collaborative approach, LPNs can significantly enhance the quality and safety of patient care. In doing so, they contribute to a cohesive and effective healthcare team where every provider has the information they need to deliver exceptional care.

1.10 Setting Priorities in Nursing Care

In nursing, the ability to prioritize patient needs effectively is essential for delivering safe, efficient, and high-quality care. LPNs often work in dynamic, fast-paced environments where competing demands require quick decision-making and thoughtful organization of tasks. By using established frameworks for prioritization and implementing practical strategies for time management, LPNs can ensure that care is both patient-centered and well-coordinated.

Frameworks for prioritizing patient needs, such as Maslow's Hierarchy of Needs and the ABC (Airway, Breathing, Circulation) model, provide structured approaches to determining which issues require immediate attention. Maslow's Hierarchy of Needs emphasizes addressing physiological and safety needs first, such as managing pain, ensuring adequate nutrition, or maintaining a safe environment. For instance, if a patient is experiencing severe pain post-surgery, this need should take precedence over routine hygiene care, as pain relief directly impacts the patient's ability to participate in recovery.

1.10.1 ABC Model

The ABC model, which stands for Airway, Breathing, and Circulation, is a foundational framework used in emergency and critical care settings to prioritize patient needs, particularly when life-threatening conditions are present. This approach ensures that the most immediate threats to a patient's survival are addressed first, providing a systematic method for identifying and managing critical issues.

Airway is the top priority because an obstructed airway prevents oxygen from reaching the lungs and the rest of the body. Without a clear airway, other interventions become irrelevant, as the patient's survival is immediately at risk. For example, if an LPN encounters a patient choking on food or experiencing severe swelling in the throat due to an allergic reaction, their first action must focus on clearing the airway. This could involve calling for advanced help, performing the Heimlich maneuver, or assisting with positioning the patient to facilitate breathing while waiting for further intervention.

Breathing follows airway management and involves ensuring that oxygen is adequately delivered to the lungs and carbon dioxide is expelled. This step is critical for sustaining life, as impaired breathing can quickly lead to hypoxia, organ damage, or cardiac arrest. An LPN might encounter a patient with labored breathing due to asthma, pneumonia, or respiratory distress syndrome. In such cases, the LPN should assess the patient's breathing rate, oxygen saturation, and effort, and take appropriate action, such as administering prescribed oxygen, assisting with positioning the patient upright to ease breathing, or initiating emergency protocols if the patient's condition deteriorates.

Circulation focuses on maintaining adequate blood flow to deliver oxygen and nutrients to tissues and organs while removing waste products. Issues with circulation can manifest as low blood pressure, poor perfusion, or abnormal heart rhythms. For instance, an LPN caring for a patient with significant blood loss following surgery must prioritize interventions to stabilize circulation. This might include monitoring vital signs for signs of shock, elevating the patient's legs to promote blood flow to vital organs, and notifying the care team for immediate action such as fluid resuscitation or blood transfusion.

The ABC model ensures that life-threatening conditions are addressed systematically and promptly, reducing the risk of complications and improving patient outcomes. It also helps LPNs stay focused in high-stress situations, guiding their actions when multiple demands compete for attention. For example, in a scenario where a patient is wheezing and struggling to breathe while another patient requires assistance with a meal, the LPN must prioritize the airway and breathing emergency over the non-urgent task. Similarly, in a code blue situation, addressing the patient's airway and breathing needs takes precedence before moving to advanced resuscitation measures.

1.10.2 Maslow's Hierarchy of Needs

Maslow's Hierarchy of Needs is a psychological theory that can be adapted to healthcare as a framework for prioritizing patient care. The hierarchy is depicted as a pyramid, with the most fundamental needs at the base and more complex, self-fulfilling needs at the top. In a clinical setting, this model helps healthcare providers, including Licensed Practical Nurses (LPNs), assess and address patient needs systematically, ensuring that essential survival needs are met before progressing to higher-level goals.

1. **Physiological Needs:** At the base of the hierarchy are physiological needs, which are critical for survival. These include essentials such as oxygen, food, water, temperature regulation, and elimination. In nursing care, these needs take the highest priority because they sustain life. For example, if a patient is dehydrated or has difficulty breathing, these issues must be addressed immediately before moving on to less urgent concerns. An LPN caring for a patient who is NPO (nothing by mouth) post-surgery might prioritize IV fluid administration to prevent dehydration and monitor the patient's oxygen levels to ensure adequate ventilation. Neglecting these fundamental needs can result in rapid deterioration of the patient's condition.
2. **Safety and Security Needs:** Once physiological needs are stabilized, the focus shifts to ensuring the patient's safety and security. This involves protecting patients from physical harm, preventing infections, and providing emotional reassurance. For instance, an LPN caring for an elderly patient at risk of falls might prioritize creating a safe environment by ensuring the call light is within reach, using bed alarms, and educating the patient about using assistive devices like walkers. Additionally, providing emotional security—such as explaining procedures in a way the patient understands—helps reduce anxiety and fosters trust in the care team.
3. **Love and Belonging Needs:** After safety is ensured, patients often seek emotional connections and a sense of belonging. In a healthcare setting, this can mean supporting relationships with family, friends, or caregivers and addressing feelings of isolation. For example, an LPN might encourage a patient recovering from a lengthy hospitalization to interact with family during visiting hours or assist with setting up a video call for those unable to visit in

person. Recognizing the importance of emotional support in recovery, the LPN might also spend time listening to the patient's concerns and ensuring they feel valued and understood.

4. **Esteem Needs:** Higher up the hierarchy are esteem needs, which include the patient's desire for respect, independence, and self-worth. In nursing care, addressing esteem needs often involves promoting the patient's autonomy and empowering them to participate in their care. For instance, an LPN might encourage a patient with limited mobility to perform parts of their hygiene routine independently, such as brushing their teeth, while offering assistance when needed. This approach not only preserves the patient's dignity but also fosters confiidence in their ability to manage aspects of their care.
5. **Self-Actualization:** At the top of the hierarchy is self-actualization, which represents the patient's ability to achieve their full potential and pursue personal goals. While this level is less immediate in the context of acute care, it becomes relevant in long-term recovery or chronic illness management. For example, an LPN working with a patient recovering from a stroke might collaborate with the healthcare team to set achievable goals for rehabilitation, such as regaining the ability to walk or return to a favorite hobby. Supporting these aspirations reinforces the patient's sense of purpose and enhances their overall quality of life.

Practical Application of Maslow's Hierarchy

In a real-world scenario, consider an LPN caring for a patient admitted with severe respiratory distress. The immediate focus would be on addressing the patient's physiological needs by ensuring adequate oxygenation and stabilizing their breathing. Once the patient's condition is stable, the LPN would turn to safety needs, such as monitoring for signs of infection and preventing falls in the hospital room. As the patient recovers, the LPN might facilitate visits from family members to address emotional support and belonging, encourage small acts of independence like self-feeding to boost esteem, and eventually help the patient set goals for continued recovery at home, supporting self-actualization.

1.11 Clarifying and Confirming Patient Consent

Clarifying and confirming patient consent is a critical responsibility for nurses, ensuring that patients fully understand their rights and the implications of the care they receive. While obtaining informed consent is typically the physician's legal duty, nurses, particularly LPNs, play a vital role in facilitating this process by educating patients, addressing their concerns, and confirming their understanding. This responsibility not only protects patients' autonomy but also supports ethical, patient-centered care.

1.11.1 The Nurse's Role in the Informed Consent Process

Informed consent is the process through which a patient voluntarily agrees to undergo a medical procedure or treatment after being provided with adequate information about its risks, benefits, alternatives, and potential outcomes. The nurse's role involves ensuring that the patient has genuinely understood this information and is making an informed decision free from coercion or undue pressure.

For example, when a patient is scheduled for surgery, the physician typically explains the procedure and obtains written consent. However, the nurse may then follow up by asking the patient questions to confirm their understanding. If the patient appears uncertain or expresses confusion about the procedure, the nurse can clarify basic points and, if needed, notify the physician to provide further explanation. The nurse acts as a bridge between the patient and the healthcare team, ensuring transparency and comprehension.

Additionally, nurses often witness the patient signing the consent form, confirming that the patient was in a clear state of mind, not under the influence of sedatives or other impairments, and that the consent was given voluntarily. For instance, if a patient is heavily sedated before surgery, the nurse should postpone signing and raise the issue with the care team, as valid consent cannot be obtained under such circumstances.

1.11.2 Strategies to Ensure Patients Understand Procedures and Risks

Effective communication is at the heart of ensuring patients understand the information presented to them. Nurses must use clear, straightforward language when discussing procedures, avoiding medical jargon that may confuse or overwhelm the patient. For example, instead of saying, "You'll undergo an angioplasty to address your arterial occlusion," a nurse might explain, "You'll have a procedure to open a blocked blood vessel in your heart to improve blood flow."

Active listening is another essential strategy. Nurses should encourage patients to ask questions and express any concerns they may have. This can be achieved by asking open-ended questions, such as, "Can you tell me in your own words what the doctor explained about the procedure?" This approach allows the nurse to identify gaps in the patient's understanding and address them promptly.

Visual aids and written materials can also enhance understanding. For example, a nurse explaining a colonoscopy might use diagrams to show the patient what the procedure involves and provide a brochure outlining the preparation steps and what to expect during recovery. These tools reinforce verbal explanations and serve as references for the patient after the conversation.

Cultural and linguistic considerations are critical when confirming consent. For patients who speak a different language, professional medical interpreters should be used to ensure that information is conveyed accurately. Relying on family members as interpreters can lead to miscommunication or omissions, particularly with sensitive or complex information. For example, a patient who doesn't fully understand the risks of a chemotherapy regimen due to a language barrier might hesitate to ask questions. By involving a professional interpreter, the nurse ensures that the patient receives all necessary information to make an informed decision.

Nonverbal cues can also provide insight into a patient's level of understanding. A patient who appears confused or hesitant may require further clarification, even if they initially express agreement. Nurses should observe these cues and proactively ask follow-up questions to confirm comprehension.

1.11.3 Addressing Challenges in the Consent Process

In some cases, patients may be reluctant to consent due to fear, anxiety, or a lack of trust in the healthcare system. Nurses can address these challenges by building rapport, expressing empathy, and creating a supportive environment where patients feel comfortable voicing their concerns. For instance, if a patient is afraid of potential side effects from a surgery, the nurse might validate their feelings by saying, "I understand that you're worried about this procedure. Let's go over the risks again, and I can help answer any questions you have." This reassurance can empower patients to make more confident, informed decisions.

For patients with cognitive impairments or diminished decision-making capacity, obtaining consent may involve additional steps, such as consulting a legally authorized representative. In such situations, the nurse must ensure that the representative has all the necessary information to make an informed decision on behalf of the patient.

1.12 Staying Within Legal Boundaries of Practice

Understanding the legal requirements for practical nursing licensure, differentiating it from certifications, and adhering to the state-mandated scope of practice are essential components of competent and ethical nursing care.

Practical nursing licensure is a state-mandated requirement that demonstrates a nurse's competency to provide safe and effective care. Each state's board of nursing establishes the specific requirements for obtaining and maintaining an LPN license, including completion of an accredited nursing program and passing the NCLEX-PN exam. Licensure serves as a legal authorization to practice nursing and ensures that individuals meet standardized educational and clinical training benchmarks. For example, a nurse cannot administer medications, perform wound care, or engage in patient education without a valid license, as these activities require demonstrated knowledge and adherence to professional standards.

Licensure is a legal safeguard for patients and the healthcare system, providing assurance that licensed professionals are adequately trained and competent to perform their duties. Practicing without a valid license is not only illegal but also poses significant risks to patients and can result in severe penalties, including fines, suspension, or permanent revocation of the right to practice.

While nursing licensure is a legal requirement to practice, nursing certifications are voluntary credentials that demonstrate expertise in specific areas of care. Certifications, such as those in IV therapy, gerontology, or wound care, enable LPNs to specialize and enhance their knowledge and skills in focused areas, but they do not replace the need for licensure. For instance, an LPN with a certification in wound care may have advanced training in managing complex wounds, but they must still hold a valid license to legally perform any nursing duties.

The legal distinction between licensure and certification is crucial. Licensure is a regulatory requirement governed by state boards, while certifications are optional credentials often granted by professional organizations. A nurse practicing without licensure is violating state laws and subject to legal consequences, whereas a nurse without certification is simply limited in their ability to specialize. For example, an LPN cannot legally provide patient care even with multiple certifications unless they hold a current and active nursing license.

Each state's nurse practice act defines the scope of practice for LPNs, outlining the tasks and responsibilities they are legally permitted to perform. Adhering to these regulations is critical to staying within legal boundaries. For instance, most states allow LPNs to administer medications, monitor patient conditions, and perform basic nursing interventions under the supervision of a registered nurse (RN) or physician. However, certain advanced procedures, such as initiating intravenous therapy or interpreting diagnostic tests, may require additional certification or be outside the LPN's scope altogether.

Practicing beyond the legal scope of practice can lead to serious consequences, including harm to patients, disciplinary actions, or legal liability. For example, if an LPN independently performs a task reserved for an RN, such as developing a comprehensive nursing care plan, they may face allegations of unprofessional conduct or malpractice. It is essential for LPNs to familiarize themselves with their state's nurse practice act and seek guidance when uncertain about their responsibilities.

Certifications can significantly enhance an LPN's ability to specialize within their scope of practice. For example:

- An LPN with a certification in IV therapy may gain advanced skills in inserting and maintaining intravenous lines, allowing them to contribute more effectively in settings like oncology or emergency care. However, this certification does not expand the LPN's scope to include tasks reserved for RNs, such as initiating certain types of infusions without supervision.

- A gerontology certification equips an LPN with specialized knowledge about the aging process, enabling them to provide tailored care to elderly patients. This specialization enhances their practice but still requires adherence to the legal boundaries of their license.

To ensure they remain within legal boundaries, LPNs must prioritize continuing education, stay informed about changes to state regulations, and seek clarification when in doubt. For example, if a healthcare facility introduces new protocols involving advanced technology, the LPN should verify whether performing related tasks is within their scope and, if necessary, pursue additional training or certifications.

Additionally, LPNs should collaborate with supervisors and colleagues to uphold safe practices. For instance, if an LPN is asked to perform a task they believe is outside their scope, such as independently assessing a complex wound, they should decline and refer the request to an RN or physician. This approach not only protects the nurse from legal repercussions but also ensures patient safety.

1.13 Collecting and Documenting Patient Data

The accurate collection and documentation of patient data are fundamental to delivering effective, safe, and patient-centered care. Documentation serves as the primary means of communication among healthcare providers, ensuring that all members of the team have access to the necessary information to make informed decisions about patient care. Licensed LPNs play a vital role in this process, contributing to the creation of a complete and reliable medical record. Understanding the legal, professional, and practical aspects of documentation is essential for maintaining accountability, supporting continuity of care, and improving patient outcomes.

Thorough and accurate data collection forms the foundation of effective patient care. Information such as vital signs, symptoms, medication administration, and patient responses to interventions must be recorded promptly and precisely. This data enables healthcare providers to monitor progress, identify trends, and adjust care plans as needed. For instance, if an LPN documents a patient's steadily increasing blood pressure over several shifts, this information alerts the team to a potential complication requiring intervention.

Accurate documentation also enhances patient safety. For example, when a nurse records a medication administration, including the time, dose, and patient's reaction, it ensures that subsequent providers are aware of any potential side effects or interactions. Errors or omissions in documentation, such as failing to note a patient's allergy to penicillin, can lead to serious consequences, including adverse reactions or harm.

Every member of the healthcare team is responsible for documenting the care they personally provide. LPNs must ensure that their entries reflect their direct observations and actions, avoiding assumptions or documenting on behalf of others. For example, if an unlicensed assistive personnel (UAP) reports a patient's temperature, the UAP is responsible for documenting this data, while the LPN verifies its accuracy and includes it in their broader assessment as needed. Similarly, RNs document activities such as care plan updates or the evaluation of patient outcomes, while LPNs focus on implementing prescribed care and monitoring patient responses. This shared responsibility promotes accuracy and accountability across the team.

Documentation is not only a professional obligation but also a legal requirement. Medical records serve as legal documents that may be referenced in court cases, audits, or investigations. Accurate, timely, and legible entries protect both the nurse and the healthcare organization by demonstrating adherence to standards of care. Each entry must include the date, time, and the nurse's signature or electronic authentication, verifying that the information is truthful and complete.

For example, if a patient develops a pressure ulcer, comprehensive documentation of the skin assessment, preventive measures, and care provided demonstrates that the nurse took appropriate actions to prevent harm. Omitting such details or falsifying records—such as documenting care that was not actually provided—can lead to legal liability, disciplinary action, or loss of licensure.

1.13.1 Comparison of Medical Record Systems

Medical record systems, such as problem-oriented medical records (POMR) and source-oriented medical records (SOMR), provide structured approaches to organizing patient information:

- **Problem-Oriented Medical Records (POMR):** In this system, documentation is organized around the patient's specific problems, with sections for a database, problem list, care plan, and progress notes. This structure fosters a holistic approach to care, as it allows providers to see all information related to a particular issue in one place. For example, if a patient is admitted for heart failure, the POMR organizes data such as diagnostic tests, medications, and interventions under the heart failure category, making it easier to track progress and outcomes.
- **Source-Oriented Medical Records (SOMR):** SOMR organizes information by discipline, with separate sections for nursing notes, physician orders, lab results, and other categories. While this system simplifies finding specific types of information, it can make it harder to view the overall picture of a patient's care. For instance, a nurse documenting in the nursing section might note a patient's pain level, while the physician's section includes related treatment orders, requiring providers to cross-reference multiple areas.

Both systems have their advantages, and nurses must adapt to the documentation system used by their facility while ensuring thorough and accurate entries.

Examples of Documentation Formats

- **SOAP Notes:** SOAP (Subjective, Objective, Assessment, Plan) is a common format for documenting progress notes. For example, an LPN documenting a patient's postoperative pain might write:
  - *Subjective:* "Patient reports pain as 7/10 in the lower abdomen."
  - *Objective:* "Surgical site appears clean and dry; no redness or swelling observed."
  - *Assessment:* "Pain likely related to surgical recovery."
  - *Plan:* "Administer prescribed pain medication and monitor response."
- **Charting by Exception:** This method focuses on documenting deviations from normal findings or expected outcomes. For instance, an LPN might note: "Patient reports increased shortness of breath with mild wheezing heard on auscultation; oxygen saturation 88%. Physician notified." Routine care, such as vital signs within normal limits, is assumed and not recorded.

1.13.2 Interdisciplinary Progress Notes

Interdisciplinary progress notes are a crucial tool for fostering effective communication and collaboration among healthcare providers. By consolidating input from multiple disciplines, these notes create a unified record that provides a comprehensive view of the patient's condition and care plan. This holistic approach ensures that every member of the healthcare team is informed of the patient's progress, interventions, and any changes to the plan of care, promoting seamless and coordinated care delivery.

For example, a physical therapist documenting progress in a patient's mobility might note increased strength and endurance during walking exercises. At the same time, an LPN could record observations about pain management interventions, such as the patient's response to prescribed medication before physical therapy sessions. Similarly, a dietitian may document improvements in nutritional intake, noting that the patient is tolerating a specific diet and has gained weight after addressing previous gastrointestinal concerns. These contributions, when documented in a single, accessible location, enable the team to assess the patient's overall progress and adjust care plans as needed.

Interdisciplinary notes also enhance the quality of patient care by minimizing redundancy and reducing the risk of miscommunication. For instance, a nurse may reference a speech therapist's notes about a patient's difficulty swallowing when planning medication administration, ensuring that pills are crushed or liquid formulations are used. Additionally, these notes provide continuity of care across shifts and between providers. When a new team member reviews the record, they can quickly understand the patient's status and the interventions already in place, allowing for informed decision-making without delays.

By consolidating information from various perspectives, interdisciplinary progress notes support a patient-centered approach to care. They ensure that all aspects of the patient's needs—physical, emotional, nutritional, and more—are addressed collaboratively. This integrated documentation not only improves patient outcomes but also strengthens the teamwork and communication essential to delivering high-quality, coordinated healthcare.

1.13.3 Scenarios Demonstrating Proper Documentation Practices

Medication Administration

Accurate documentation of medication administration is critical for ensuring patient safety, continuity of care, and evaluating the effectiveness of treatments. For example, an LPN administering insulin to a patient with diabetes would document specific details, including the type of insulin (e.g., rapid-acting or long-acting), the exact dose given, the time of administration, and the injection site (e.g., left abdomen or right thigh). This entry should also include any pre- and post-administration observations, such as the patient's blood glucose level and their response to the medication. For instance, if the patient's pre-dose blood sugar was 250 mg/dL and dropped to 140 mg/dL after insulin administration, this outcome should be recorded to provide a clear picture of the medication's effectiveness. If adverse reactions occur, such as dizziness or confusion, these must also be documented, along with the actions taken to address them. Thorough documentation ensures that subsequent care providers can build on this information and adjust treatment plans as needed.

Reporting a Fall

When a patient experiences a fall, detailed and objective documentation is essential for ensuring patient safety and demonstrating adherence to protocols. For example, if a patient is found sitting on the floor after tripping over bed linens, the LPN should document the exact time and circumstances of the incident, such as: "Patient found sitting on floor at 11:00 AM, reports tripping over bed linens while getting out of bed. No visible injuries noted. Patient alert and oriented to person, place, and time. Physician and supervisor notified. Fall risk interventions reinforced, including placement of call light within reach and removal of hazards." This entry captures the facts without speculation or blame, highlighting the nurse's immediate actions and communication with the care team. Such documentation serves as a legal safeguard and supports quality improvement initiatives by identifying potential environmental or procedural factors contributing to falls.

Wound Care Assessment

Wound care requires meticulous documentation to track healing progress and ensure continuity of care. For example, when dressing a patient's pressure ulcer, an LPN should record the wound's location, size (e.g., length, width, and depth), the presence and amount of drainage (e.g., serous, purulent), and the wound's appearance (e.g., granulating tissue, redness, or necrosis). Additionally, the type of dressing applied and the patient's tolerance to the procedure should be documented.

An entry might read: "Dressed Stage 2 pressure ulcer on sacrum at 10:00 AM. Wound measures 3 cm x 2 cm x 0.5 cm, with moderate serous drainage. Edges appear pink with granulation tissue present; no signs of infection noted. Applied hydrocolloid dressing. Patient tolerated procedure without discomfort and verbalized understanding of wound care instructions." This level of detail not only supports ongoing monitoring but also provides a clear record for evaluation by other team members, such as wound care specialists or physicians.

Additional Considerations for Documentation Scenarios

1. **Monitoring Pain Management:** If an LPN administers an analgesic for post-operative pain, they should document the patient's pain level before and after the medication, using a standard pain scale (e.g., 7/10 before, 3/10 one hour after). This ensures that pain relief measures are evaluated for effectiveness and provides evidence of adherence to the care plan.
2. **Managing Infections:** If a patient exhibits signs of infection, such as a fever or elevated white blood cell count, the LPN should document these findings, notify the physician, and record any subsequent actions, such as obtaining a blood culture or administering prescribed antibiotics.
3. **Addressing Patient Complaints:** If a patient complains of dizziness after receiving a new medication, the LPN should document the complaint, assess vital signs, and report the findings to the care team. For example: "Patient reports dizziness at 9:00 AM following administration of antihypertensive medication. Blood pressure measured at 90/60 mmHg. Physician notified and order received to hold next dose and monitor vitals hourly."

1.14 Coordinating Referrals for Comprehensive Care

Coordinating referrals to appropriate services is a vital aspect of nursing care that ensures patients receive comprehensive and specialized support beyond the immediate scope of bedside care. LPNs play an important role in facilitating referrals, acting as a bridge between patients, families, and a variety of healthcare services. Proper coordination of referrals helps maintain continuity of care, supports patient recovery, and addresses long-term health and social needs.

The referral process begins with a comprehensive assessment of the patient's needs, identifying areas that require additional expertise or support beyond what the immediate care team can provide. These needs might include specialized medical care, rehabilitation services, social support, or access to community-based programs. For instance, a patient recovering from a stroke may require a multifaceted approach involving physical therapy to restore mobility, speech therapy to address communication challenges, and social services to help adapt their home environment for safety and accessibility. These referrals ensure that the patient receives holistic care tailored to their unique circumstances.

LPNs play a pivotal role in coordinating referrals by collaborating with the healthcare team to determine the most appropriate services based on the patient's condition, treatment plan, and personal goals. This collaboration often involves consulting with registered nurses (RNs), physicians, and case managers to develop a comprehensive understanding of the patient's overall health status and specific needs. LPNs assist in collecting essential information such as medical history, current diagnoses, and any relevant clinical notes or test results. This documentation ensures that the receiving provider or service has a complete picture of the patient's condition, enabling them to deliver targeted and effective care.

Education is another critical component of the referral process. LPNs work closely with patients and their families to explain the purpose of the referral, outlining how the recommended service will contribute to their overall care and recovery. For example, when referring a patient with chronic kidney disease to a nephrologist, the LPN might explain how specialized care will help manage their condition, prevent complications, and improve their quality of life. This education empowers patients to engage actively in their care, increasing the likelihood of compliance with follow-up appointments and interventions.

Effective communication is essential throughout the referral process to ensure a smooth transition to the recommended service. LPNs may need to contact external providers, schedule appointments, and coordinate logistical details such as transportation or financial assistance. For example, if a patient with diabetes requires ongoing dietary counseling, the LPN might identify a local registered dietitian, schedule an initial consultation, and provide the patient with key details, including the time and location of the appointment, any required preparation, and what to expect during the visit. Additionally, the LPN might connect the patient with community resources to address barriers, such as transportation services or insurance coverage, ensuring that the referral is accessible and feasible.

1.14.1 Scenarios Illustrating Referrals Enhancing Continuity of Care

1. **Post-Hospitalization Rehabilitation**

   Consider a patient discharged after a hip replacement surgery. The LPN identifies that the patient requires physical therapy to regain mobility and occupational therapy to learn how to perform daily activities safely at home. The LPN collaborates with the discharge planner to arrange these referrals, ensuring that the patient's appointments are scheduled before discharge. Additionally, the LPN educates the patient on the importance of attending these sessions to prevent complications like joint stiffness or muscle weakness. By coordinating these referrals, the LPN ensures the patient has a seamless transition from hospital care to outpatient services.

2. **Management of Chronic Illness**

   A patient with newly diagnosed hypertension struggles to manage their condition despite medication. The LPN, recognizing the patient's difficulty adhering to dietary recommendations, arranges a referral to a dietitian specializing in hypertension management. The dietitian provides meal planning strategies and education on sodium intake, while the LPN follows up to assess the patient's progress and reinforce these recommendations. This collaborative effort ensures the patient receives tailored support, improving their ability to manage their condition effectively.

3. **Social Support for Vulnerable Patients**

   An elderly patient living alone is admitted for malnutrition and dehydration. The LPN identifies social factors contributing to the patient's condition, such as limited access to groceries and lack of family support. To address these needs, the LPN arranges a referral to a social worker, who connects the patient with meal delivery services and senior support programs. This coordinated approach addresses both medical and social needs, promoting the patient's overall well-being and reducing the likelihood of readmission.

4. **Specialized Care for Mental Health**

   A young adult patient admitted with anxiety and sleep disturbances requires long-term mental health support. The LPN collaborates with the healthcare team to arrange a referral to a mental health counselor and provides the patient with information on local support groups. Additionally, the LPN encourages the patient to follow through with appointments and offers reassurance about the benefits of seeking professional help. This proactive referral ensures the patient has access to resources that address their mental health needs comprehensively

Referrals play a crucial role in maintaining continuity of care, ensuring that patients receive support at every stage of their health journey. They prevent gaps in care by linking patients to specialized services, addressing needs that cannot be fully managed within the primary healthcare setting. For example, a patient recovering from a cardiac event may require coordination between a cardiologist, a physical therapist, and a pharmacist to manage their recovery effectively.

By coordinating referrals, LPNs enhance collaboration among healthcare providers, ensuring that interventions are aligned with the patient's goals and needs. This coordination fosters a holistic approach to care, addressing physical, emotional, and social aspects of health. It also empowers patients to take an active role in their care, equipping them with the resources and knowledge needed for long-term management of their conditions.

Chapter 2
Safety and Infection Control

This chapter explores essential strategies to create a secure environment for clients and healthcare providers. From understanding proper hand hygiene and personal protective equipment (PPE) to managing hazardous materials and implementing isolation protocols, the content emphasizes best practices to reduce risks. By mastering these principles, nurses can effectively safeguard clients from harm while maintaining a safe, compliant workplace.

2.1 Apply Infection Control Principles

The healthcare environment, while designed to promote healing, often involves invasive procedures, close patient proximity, and interactions with individuals who may carry infectious agents. These factors create opportunities for the spread of infections if stringent precautions are not observed.

The primary goal of infection control is to prevent the transmission of pathogens and reduce the incidence of healthcare-associated infections (HAIs). HAIs, such as catheter-associated urinary tract infections (CAUTIs), surgical site infections, and bloodstream infections, are not only costly but can also lead to prolonged hospital stays, increased morbidity, and, in severe cases, mortality. For healthcare providers, effective infection prevention safeguards their health, minimizes occupational risks, and ensures compliance with legal and professional standards.

By prioritizing infection prevention, nurses create an environment of safety and trust. Licensed Practical Nurses (LPNs) play a vital role in this effort, implementing evidence-based practices, adhering to infection control protocols, and educating patients and their families about ways to minimize infection risks. This foundational knowledge allows LPNs to address both routine and high-risk care scenarios effectively.

2.1.1 Assessing Clients' Susceptibility to Infections

Not all patients face the same risk of infection. Some populations are particularly vulnerable due to weakened immune systems, chronic conditions, or specific medical treatments. Identifying these vulnerable populations is a critical step in tailoring infection prevention strategies to individual needs.

Vulnerable Populations

Patients with neutropenia, often a result of chemotherapy, have significantly reduced white blood cell counts, making them less able to fight off infections. Similarly, individuals with Cushing's disease or those receiving corticosteroid therapy face an increased risk due to impaired immune responses. LPNs must remain vigilant in recognizing these risks, ensuring that appropriate precautions are in place to minimize exposure to pathogens.

Implementation of Specific Precautions

To safeguard immunocompromised patients, healthcare providers implement a range of targeted precautions designed to reduce infection risks while promoting recovery:

1. **Private Room Assignments:** Assigning a private room minimizes exposure to other patients who may carry infectious agents. For example, a patient undergoing chemotherapy with severe neutropenia should be placed in a private room to reduce the risk of airborne or droplet-transmitted infections from other individuals in shared spaces.
2. **Isolation Protocols:** In some cases, strict isolation is necessary to protect immunocompromised patients. For instance, reverse isolation, where healthcare staff and visitors wear protective clothing to prevent transmitting infections to the patient, is often used for individuals with extremely compromised immune systems. This protocol ensures that external contaminants do not compromise patient safety.
3. **Dietary Restrictions:** Dietary modifications can also play a significant role in infection prevention. For example, immunocompromised patients are often advised to avoid raw vegetables, which can carry bacteria that are difficult to eliminate through washing. Similarly, undercooked meats and unpasteurized dairy products should be excluded from their diets to minimize the risk of foodborne illnesses.
4. **Avoidance of Fresh Flowers and Plants:** While flowers and plants may seem innocuous, they can harbor molds and bacteria that pose a threat to immunocompromised patients. For example, a patient with neutropenia may be advised to avoid having fresh flowers in their room to eliminate potential fungal spores that could exacerbate their condition.
5. **Avoidance of Rectal Procedures:** Procedures such as rectal suppositories, enemas, or temperature measurements should be avoided in vulnerable patients due to the risk of introducing pathogens into the rectal mucosa, which can easily become a portal of entry for infections. For example, an LPN caring for a patient with Cushing's disease should opt for alternative methods to manage constipation or administer medications.

Case Example: Neutropenic Patient

Consider a patient undergoing chemotherapy for leukemia, resulting in severe neutropenia. The LPN assigns the patient to a private room and implements reverse isolation protocols. Dietary instructions are given to avoid raw produce, and family members are advised not to bring fresh flowers during visits. During medication administration, the LPN ensures that all aseptic techniques are strictly followed, avoiding any invasive rectal procedures. These steps collectively minimize the patient's exposure to infection and promote a safer recovery environment.

2.1.2 Preventing Healthcare-Associated Infections (HAIs)

Healthcare-associated infections (HAIs) represent a significant challenge in medical settings, contributing to prolonged hospital stays, increased healthcare costs, and adverse patient outcomes. As frontline caregivers, Licensed Practical Nurses (LPNs) play a critical role in preventing these infections by implementing evidence-based strategies and adhering to stringent infection control protocols. Three common HAIs—catheter-related infections, intravenous (IV) line infections, and *Clostridioides difficile (C. difficile)* infections—require particular attention due to their prevalence and potential severity.

Key HAIs to Address

1. **Catheter-Related Infections:** Indwelling urinary catheters are a leading cause of catheter-associated urinary tract infections (CAUTIs). These infections occur when bacteria enter the urinary tract through the catheter, often due to improper insertion or prolonged use. Symptoms may include fever, urinary discomfort, and cloudy or odorous urine.
2. **Intravenous (IV) Line Infections:** IV lines, especially central lines, can serve as entry points for pathogens, leading to bloodstream infections. Contamination during insertion, improper maintenance, or failure to adhere to aseptic techniques increases the risk of complications such as sepsis. Symptoms of infection may include redness or swelling at the insertion site, fever, or chills.
3. ***C. difficile* Infections:** *C. difficile* is a spore-forming bacterium that causes severe diarrhea and colitis, often in patients who have received antibiotics that disrupt normal gut flora. Transmission occurs via the fecal-oral route, often due to poor hand hygiene or contaminated surfaces in healthcare environments. Symptoms include watery diarrhea, abdominal pain, and fever.

Strategies to Prevent HAIs

1. **Minimizing Indwelling Urinary Catheter Use and Limiting Duration:** Reducing the use of urinary catheters and removing them as soon as clinically indicated are effective strategies for preventing CAUTIs. LPNs can assess daily whether a catheter remains necessary and advocate for its timely removal. For instance, if a patient recovering from surgery regains mobility and can void independently, the LPN should recommend discontinuing the catheter. When

catheters are used, following aseptic insertion techniques and maintaining a closed drainage system are crucial to minimizing infection risks.

2. **Adhering to Strict Aseptic Techniques:** Proper aseptic technique is essential for preventing IV line infections and other HAIs. During IV insertion or catheter placement, LPNs must use sterile gloves, antiseptic solutions to clean the insertion site, and sterile drapes to maintain a contaminant-free field. Additionally, regular site assessments and timely dressing changes help prevent infection. For example, an LPN caring for a patient with a central line should inspect the site daily for redness, swelling, or discharge and promptly report any signs of infection to the care team.
3. **Preventing *C. difficile* Spread:** Effective hand hygiene using soap and water—rather than alcohol-based hand sanitizers—is critical for removing C. difficile spores. Environmental cleaning with sporicidal agents ensures that surfaces, including bedrails and doorknobs, are free of contamination. LPNs should also adhere to contact precautions, such as wearing gloves and gowns when interacting with infected patients, to prevent cross-contamination. Educating patients and families about the importance of handwashing and environmental sanitation further supports infection control efforts.

2.1.3 Principles of Surgical Asepsis

Surgical asepsis, or sterile technique, involves practices designed to eliminate all microorganisms from an environment, ensuring that invasive procedures are conducted without introducing pathogens. This approach is critical for preventing HAIs during surgeries, catheter insertions, and other sterile procedures.

Creating, Maintaining, and Handling Sterile Fields

To create a sterile field, LPNs must begin with meticulous preparation, including hand hygiene, donning sterile gloves, and using sterile drapes to establish a contaminant-free area. All items within the sterile field, such as instruments and dressings, must remain sterile.

Maintaining sterility requires constant vigilance. For example:

- **Maintaining the boundary:** Items should not be placed near the edges of a sterile drape, as these areas are considered non-sterile.
- **Preventing contamination:** Avoid turning away from the sterile field, as this prevents monitoring for accidental breaches.

During procedures, LPNs must minimize unnecessary movement and conversation near the sterile field to reduce the risk of contamination from airborne particles.

Common Violations and Corrective Actions

Despite careful preparation, breaches in sterile technique can occur. Examples include:

- Touching sterile items with non-sterile gloves.
- Allowing sterile items to come into contact with contaminated surfaces.
- Placing items too close to the edge of the sterile field.

When sterility is compromised, LPNs must restart the setup to ensure patient safety. For instance, if a sterile dressing inadvertently falls off the field and contacts the floor, it must be replaced with a new sterile dressing. Attempting to reuse contaminated items can lead to serious infections.

Case Example: Central Line Dressing Change

An LPN changing the dressing of a central line must follow surgical asepsis principles. After performing hand hygiene, they gather sterile supplies, clean the site with antiseptic solution, and apply a sterile dressing without touching the adhesive side. If they accidentally brush the dressing against their sleeve, they discard it and use a new dressing to maintain sterility.

By adhering to the principles of surgical asepsis, LPNs uphold the highest standards of infection prevention, ensuring safe and effective care during invasive procedures.

2.1.4 Modes of Transmission of Infections

Understanding the modes of infection transmission is critical for implementing effective infection control measures in healthcare settings. Transmission occurs when pathogens move from a source to a susceptible host via vectors, fomites, or direct contact. By identifying these modes and implementing targeted strategies, Licensed Practical Nurses (LPNs) can minimize the risk of infections among patients and healthcare workers.

Differentiating Vectors, Fomites, and Hosts

1. **Vectors:** Vectors are living organisms, such as flies, mosquitoes, or vermin, that transmit infectious agents from one host to another. For example, mosquitoes are vectors for diseases like malaria and dengue fever, while rats can carry pathogens responsible for leptospirosis or hantavirus. In healthcare, vector control is essential to prevent outbreaks, particularly in facilities located in tropical or rural areas.
2. **Fomites:** Fomites are non-living objects or surfaces that can carry and transmit pathogens. Examples include contaminated thermometers, stethoscopes, or bed rails. These objects often serve as indirect transmission routes, particularly when healthcare workers fail to clean equipment between patient uses. For instance, an improperly disinfected blood pressure cuff can spread bacteria like *Staphylococcus aureus*.

3. **Hosts:** Hosts are individuals who harbor infectious agents and can transmit them to others. Hosts may be symptomatic, as in the case of a patient with active tuberculosis, or asymptomatic carriers, such as someone shedding *Salmonella* without showing signs of illness. Recognizing and isolating infectious hosts is crucial for preventing disease spread.

Strategies to Interrupt Transmission

1. **Pest Control:** Preventing the presence of vectors, such as flies or rodents, is essential in reducing disease transmission. Healthcare facilities should maintain strict pest control measures, including sealing entry points, using traps or insecticides, and eliminating standing water where mosquitoes breed.
2. **Environmental Sanitation:** Regular cleaning and disinfection of surfaces and equipment reduce the risk of fomite transmission. For example, high-touch areas like doorknobs, keyboards, and medical equipment should be cleaned frequently with hospital-grade disinfectants.
3. **Proper Use of Personal Protective Equipment (PPE):** PPE serves as a barrier against direct and indirect transmission. Gloves, gowns, masks, and eye protection should be used according to the level of risk, and proper donning and doffing techniques must be followed to prevent contamination. For instance, an LPN caring for a patient with *C. difficile* must wear gloves and gowns, ensuring they are discarded properly before exiting the room.

2.1.5 Transmission-Based Precautions

Transmission-based precautions are additional infection control measures implemented when patients are known or suspected to be infected with specific pathogens. These precautions vary based on the mode of transmission and include minimal PPE requirements for each scenario.

Types of Precautions and Minimal PPE Requirements

1. **Contact Precautions:** Used for infections transmitted through direct or indirect contact with contaminated surfaces or bodily fluids, such as *C. difficile* or MRSA.

   - **PPE:** Gloves and gowns.
   - *Example:* An LPN caring for a patient with a wound infection wears gloves and a gown, ensuring hand hygiene before and after patient interaction.

2. **Droplet Precautions:** Applied for infections spread through respiratory droplets, such as influenza or pertussis.

   - **PPE:** A face mask.
   - *Example:* When caring for a patient with suspected influenza, the LPN wears a surgical mask and maintains a distance of at least six feet when possible.

3. **Airborne Precautions:** Necessary for infections transmitted through airborne particles, such as tuberculosis or measles.
   - **PPE:** HEPA mask, gown, gloves, and use of a negative pressure room.
   - *Example:* A patient with active tuberculosis is placed in a negative pressure room, and the LPN wears a fitted N95 respirator mask while providing care.

Examples of Implementing Precautions

1. **Negative Pressure Rooms:** Patients with airborne infections are isolated in rooms with specialized ventilation systems that prevent contaminated air from escaping. An LPN caring for a patient with tuberculosis ensures the door remains closed and verifies that the negative pressure system is functioning properly.
2. **Room Assignments:** Assigning patients based on their infection status is critical. For example, a patient with C. difficile should not share a room with an immunocompromised individual to prevent cross-contamination.

2.1.6 Teaching Strategies for Infection Control

Education and training are vital for ensuring healthcare staff consistently adhere to infection control protocols. LPNs can contribute by providing demonstrations and reinforcing best practices among colleagues and patients.

1. **Demonstrations on Proper PPE Usage and Disposal:** Demonstrations on how to don (put on) and doff (remove) PPE correctly reduce the risk of contamination. For example, LPNs might conduct in-service training showing staff how to remove gloves without touching the contaminated exterior and how to safely discard used masks.
2. **Reinforcement of Compliance with Infection Control Protocols:** Regular reminders and audits ensure adherence to protocols. For instance, LPNs can emphasize the importance of hand hygiene before and after patient contact and use visual aids or posters in staff areas to reinforce these practices.

Case Example: Education on PPE

During a staff meeting, an LPN observes improper PPE removal techniques among team members. To address this, they organize a hands-on training session, demonstrating step-by-step procedures for safely removing gloves, masks, and gowns. This ensures compliance and enhances safety for both staff and patients.

2.1.7 Evidence-Based Practices for Infection Prevention

Adopting evidence-based practices is crucial for minimizing infection risks and ensuring patient safety in both routine and high-risk care settings. These practices are informed by research and clinical guidelines, enabling nurses to provide effective care while preventing the transmission of pathogens. Licensed Practical Nurses (LPNs) play an essential role in implementing these strategies, ensuring compliance among staff, and educating patients about infection prevention.

Routine and High-Risk Care Settings

1. **Hand Hygiene:** Hand hygiene is the cornerstone of infection prevention and is one of the most effective ways to reduce healthcare-associated infections (HAIs). LPNs must practice proper handwashing techniques using soap and water or alcohol-based hand sanitizers, depending on the situation. For example, soap and water are mandatory when dealing with *Clostridioides difficile* spores, while hand sanitizers may suffice in other scenarios. Hand hygiene must be performed:

    - Before and after patient contact.
    - Before aseptic procedures.
    - After contact with bodily fluids or contaminated surfaces.
    - After removing gloves.

2. **Appropriate PPE Use:** Proper selection, donning, and doffing of personal protective equipment (PPE) are vital to creating a barrier between the nurse and potential sources of infection. For instance, gloves and gowns are necessary when dealing with patients under contact precautions, while an N95 respirator is required for airborne precautions. Ensuring that PPE fits correctly and is used according to protocol reduces exposure risks.
3. **Maintaining Sterile Techniques:** Sterile techniques are critical for preventing contamination during procedures such as catheter insertions, wound dressing changes, and surgeries. This includes creating and maintaining sterile fields, avoiding unnecessary movements that could introduce airborne contaminants, and restarting the procedure if sterility is compromised. For example, when inserting a Foley catheter, the LPN ensures that all supplies remain sterile and avoids touching the catheter tip with non-sterile gloves or surfaces.

Nurse's Role in Identifying Ineffective Practices

LPNs are frontline advocates for best practices and must identify and address ineffective or outdated infection prevention methods. For example, unnecessary granulocyte transfusions, once believed to prevent infections in immunocompromised patients, are now considered ineffective in many cases. LPNs should question practices that lack evidence and collaborate with the healthcare team to adopt current guidelines. Similarly, an LPN noticing frequent breaches in hand hygiene protocols among staff might organize reminders or training sessions to reinforce compliance.

Scenarios and Teaching Tools to Reinforce Protocols

Practical scenarios and teaching tools are effective in training healthcare workers and patients. For instance:

- *Scenario:* During a simulated wound dressing change, staff practice identifying breaches in sterile technique, such as a gloved hand touching a non-sterile object. Feedback is provided to improve performance.
- *Teaching Tools:* Visual aids like posters illustrating the steps of hand hygiene or videos demonstrating correct PPE usage can serve as reminders in high-traffic areas.

2.1.8 Infection Control in Wound Care

Proper wound care is an integral part of infection prevention, ensuring that wounds heal efficiently while minimizing the risk of complications. LPNs are often responsible for performing wound care, which requires a thorough understanding of aseptic techniques and appropriate interventions.

1. **Proper Wound Care Techniques**
   - **Irrigation to Cleanse Wounds:** Wound irrigation is a critical step to remove debris, bacteria, and exudate from the wound bed, promoting a clean environment for healing. LPNs use sterile saline or prescribed solutions and ensure that the irrigation flows from the cleanest to the dirtiest area to prevent contamination. For instance, a chronic leg ulcer is irrigated with a syringe and catheter tip, maintaining sterile technique throughout.
   - **Facilitating Healing with Medication Applications:** After cleansing, medications such as antimicrobial ointments or dressings infused with silver can be applied to reduce bacterial load and promote healing. LPNs ensure these medications are applied evenly and that the wound is covered with an appropriate dressing to maintain a moist, protective environment.

2. **Examples to Demonstrate Wound Care Protocols**
   - **Scenario 1 - Managing a Surgical Wound:** An LPN caring for a post-operative patient observes slight redness around a surgical incision. Using sterile gloves, the LPN irrigates the wound with sterile saline, applies an antimicrobial dressing, and documents the findings. The LPN educates the patient on monitoring for signs of infection, such as increased redness, swelling, or drainage.
   - **Scenario 2 - Dressing a Diabetic Foot Ulcer** For a patient with a diabetic foot ulcer, the LPN uses sterile technique to remove the old dressing, irrigates the wound with a prescribed solution, and applies a hydrocolloid dressing. The LPN ensures that all contaminated materials are disposed of properly and educates the patient on offloading pressure from the wound to support healing.

2.2 Use Transfer Assistive Devices Safely

Transfer devices reduce the risk of injuries, such as strains or falls, while promoting comfort and dignity for patients who may have limited mobility. Employing these tools effectively requires proper training, adherence to safety protocols, and a patient-centered approach.

Transfer assistive devices include a variety of tools designed to aid in the safe movement of patients. These devices are used in scenarios such as transferring a patient from a bed to a wheelchair, repositioning in a bed, or assisting with standing and walking. Common devices include:

1. **Transfer Belts:** Also known as **gait belts**, transfer belts are worn around the patient's waist to provide caregivers with a secure grip during transfers. They are particularly useful for patients with some mobility who require minimal to moderate assistance.
2. **Mechanical Lifts:** Mechanical lifts, such as hydraulic or electric Hoyer lifts, are designed for patients with limited or no mobility. These devices use slings to lift and transfer patients from one surface to another, such as from a bed to a wheelchair.
3. **Slide Boards:** Slide boards are used for lateral transfers, such as moving a patient from a wheelchair to a bed. They reduce friction and allow for smoother, safer transitions.
4. **Sit-to-Stand Devices:** These devices assist patients who can bear some weight but need support transitioning from sitting to standing positions.

2.2.1 Steps for Safe Use of Transfer Assistive Devices

1. **Assess the Patient's Needs and Abilities**
   Before using a transfer device, evaluate the patient's condition, mobility level, weight, and any specific limitations. For example, a patient recovering from a stroke may require a transfer belt for walking assistance, while a non-ambulatory patient may need a mechanical lift.

2. **Prepare the Environment**
   Ensure the transfer area is free of obstacles, such as clutter, cords, or uneven surfaces. Lock the wheels of beds or wheelchairs to prevent movement during the transfer. For instance, when using a slide board to transfer a patient from a wheelchair to a bed, ensure both surfaces are at similar heights and securely positioned.

3. **Communicate with the Patient**
   Explain the transfer process to the patient, providing clear instructions and reassurance. For example: "I'm going to use this transfer belt to help you stand and move to the wheelchair. Please hold onto the armrest once you're seated." This promotes cooperation and reduces anxiety.

4. **Use Proper Body Mechanics**
   Caregivers must prioritize their own safety by using proper body mechanics. Keep the back straight, bend at the knees, and use leg muscles for lifting rather than the back. Maintain a wide base of support and avoid twisting movements.

5. **Operate the Device Correctly**
   Follow the manufacturer's instructions for the specific device. For example:

   - **Transfer Belt:** Secure the belt snugly around the patient's waist, ensuring it is not too tight or positioned over fragile areas. Stand close to the patient and use an underhand grip to provide steady support.
   - **Mechanical Lift:** Position the sling correctly under the patient, ensuring even weight distribution. Operate the lift slowly and steadily, communicating with the patient throughout the process to ensure comfort.

6. **Monitor the Patient**
   Observe the patient for signs of discomfort, dizziness, or fear during the transfer. If the patient appears unstable or expresses distress, pause the transfer and reassess the approach.

Examples of Safe Use of Transfer Devices

1. **Using a Transfer Belt for Assisted Ambulation**
   A patient recovering from hip surgery requires assistance walking to the bathroom. The LPN secures a transfer belt around the patient's waist, providing a stable grip to guide them while walking. The LPN maintains a supportive stance, staying close to the patient to prevent falls, and removes the belt once the patient is seated securely.

2. **Using a Mechanical Lift for Bed-to-Wheelchair Transfer**
   An immobile patient with advanced arthritis needs to be moved from bed to a wheelchair. The LPN positions the sling under the patient, ensuring it supports the back and legs evenly. Using the mechanical lift, the patient is gently lifted and transferred to the wheelchair, ensuring their comfort and safety throughout the process.

3. **Repositioning with a Slide Board**
   A patient with partial paralysis needs to move from a wheelchair to a bed. The LPN places the slide board under the patient's thighs and uses a gentle push-pull motion to guide the patient onto the bed, minimizing strain for both the caregiver and the patient.

Benefits of Proper Use of Transfer Devices

- **Prevents Injuries:** Reduces strain on caregivers' backs and minimizes the risk of patient falls.
- **Promotes Dignity:** Ensures patients are moved safely and comfortably, preserving their sense of independence and respect.
- **Improves Efficiency:** Streamlines transfers, saving time while maintaining safety and reducing the need for additional staff assistance.

2.3 Evaluate Client Care Orders

Evaluating client care orders is a critical responsibility for Licensed Practical Nurses (LPNs) to ensure that treatments and interventions are accurate, safe, and aligned with the LPN's scope of practice. Proper review and verification of healthcare provider instructions not only safeguard patient well-being but also reinforce the integrity of collaborative care within the healthcare team. LPNs must remain vigilant in identifying tasks that are appropriate for their role while recognizing when to escalate responsibilities to Registered Nurses (RNs) or other team members. Understanding legal and professional boundaries is essential in maintaining compliance with nursing standards and providing high-quality care.

When receiving care orders, LPNs must ensure that instructions are clear, accurate, and within their scope of practice. This involves confirming the following:

- **Clarity:** Orders must be legible, specific, and unambiguous. For instance, an order for medication should include the drug name, dose, route, and timing. If an order lacks detail, the LPN must seek clarification from the prescribing provider.
- **Safety:** Orders must align with best practices and the patient's condition. For example, a dose of insulin that seems unusually high for a patient's blood glucose level warrants verification to prevent harm.
- **Scope of Practice:** LPNs must evaluate whether the task is within their legal scope. For instance, an LPN can administer most medications but is typically not authorized to administer chemotherapy or initiate blood transfusions.

2.3.1 Tasks Appropriate for LPNs

Licensed Practical Nurses (LPNs) play a critical role in delivering hands-on patient care through tasks that require technical expertise, precision, and adherence to safety protocols. Their scope of practice is defined by state regulations and facility policies, allowing them to perform a wide range of essential duties. Below are detailed examples of tasks within an LPN's scope and the responsibilities involved in executing these tasks effectively.

Inserting and Managing Foley Catheters

LPNs are frequently tasked with inserting and maintaining urinary catheters, ensuring both patient comfort and infection prevention.

- **Insertion:** LPNs use sterile techniques to insert catheters, minimizing the risk of introducing pathogens. Proper patient positioning, effective communication, and skillful handling of equipment are vital to ensure a smooth and safe procedure.
- **Management:** Once the catheter is in place, LPNs monitor for complications such as urinary tract infections (UTIs) or blockages. They check for signs of infection, such as cloudy urine or foul odors, and promptly report abnormalities to the healthcare team.

- **Documentation:** Recording the time of insertion, type and size of the catheter, urine output, and any observed abnormalities ensures accurate tracking and continuity of care.

Example: A patient recovering from surgery is unable to void independently. The LPN inserts a Foley catheter using aseptic technique, records the urine output every two hours, and monitors for signs of infection.

Obtaining Specimens

LPNs play an integral role in collecting diagnostic specimens such as blood, urine, sputum, and wound cultures. Accurate specimen collection contributes to timely and reliable diagnostic outcomes.

- **Blood Specimen Collection:** LPNs trained in phlebotomy can draw blood samples, ensuring that proper venipuncture techniques are used to prevent hemolysis and patient discomfort.
- **Urine Specimens:** For a clean-catch sample, the LPN educates the patient on proper technique to avoid contamination. In catheterized patients, the LPN collects the sample directly from the catheter port using sterile equipment.
- **Wound Cultures:** When collecting wound cultures, LPNs clean the wound per protocol before obtaining the sample to avoid cross-contamination and ensure accurate results.

Example: A patient with a suspected urinary tract infection requires a urine sample. The LPN collects the sample, labels it with the correct patient information, and delivers it to the lab promptly.

Administering Medications

Medication administration is a key responsibility for LPNs, requiring thorough knowledge of pharmacology and adherence to safety protocols. The scope of medication administration varies by state and facility policy but typically includes:

- **Oral Medications:** Administering tablets, capsules, and liquid medications while monitoring for effectiveness and potential side effects.
- **Subcutaneous and Intramuscular Injections:** LPNs administer insulin, vaccines, and other medications via these routes, ensuring correct dosage and injection site rotation to prevent complications like lipodystrophy.
- **Intravenous Medications:** Depending on state regulations, LPNs may administer certain IV medications. However, IV push medications or complex infusions, such as chemotherapy, are usually reserved for RNs.

Example: A patient with diabetes requires insulin before meals. The LPN verifies the order, checks the patient's blood glucose level, prepares the correct insulin dose, and administers the injection using proper technique.

Basic Wound Care and Dressing Changes

LPNs are often responsible for managing wounds that do not require advanced interventions. This includes cleaning, dressing, and monitoring wounds for signs of infection or delayed healing.

- **Wound Cleaning:** LPNs use antiseptic solutions to clean wounds, following aseptic or sterile techniques as appropriate.
- **Dressing Application:** Applying appropriate dressings, such as gauze or hydrocolloid, based on the care plan.
- **Observation:** Documenting wound size, color, drainage, and other findings to aid in evaluating the effectiveness of treatment.

Example: An LPN performs a dressing change for a patient with a surgical incision, noting decreased redness and minimal serous drainage, and communicates these findings to the RN.

Monitoring Vital Signs and Patient Status

LPNs frequently monitor and record vital signs, such as blood pressure, heart rate, respiratory rate, and temperature, to assess patient stability.

- **Routine Monitoring:** Regular checks during routine care to identify early signs of deterioration.
- **Specialized Monitoring:** For patients with specific conditions, such as hypertension or fever, LPNs may take frequent readings to guide treatment decisions.

Example: An LPN checks the vital signs of a patient receiving IV antibiotics for pneumonia, noting a drop in temperature and improved oxygen saturation, indicating a positive response to treatment.

Performing Basic Respiratory Care

LPNs can provide basic respiratory interventions to support patients with compromised breathing.

- **Oxygen Therapy:** Setting up and monitoring oxygen delivery systems, such as nasal cannulas or face masks.
- **Nebulizer Treatments:** Administering prescribed medications via nebulizer and evaluating the patient's response.

Example: An LPN administers a bronchodilator treatment to a patient with asthma and observes improved breath sounds post-treatment.

Assisting with Feeding Tubes

LPNs manage enteral feeding for patients who are unable to eat orally.

- **Tube Feedings:** Administering prescribed feeding solutions via nasogastric (NG) or percutaneous endoscopic gastrostomy (PEG) tubes.
- **Monitoring for Complications:** Checking for signs of aspiration, tube displacement, or feeding intolerance, such as nausea or abdominal distension.

> *Example:* An LPN administers a feeding through a PEG tube and checks for residual volume to ensure the patient is tolerating the nutrition.

Providing Emotional Support and Education

LPNs often serve as a source of emotional support for patients and families, explaining procedures and answering questions to reduce anxiety.

- **Patient Education:** Teaching patients about medication regimens, wound care, or mobility exercises.
- **Emotional Reassurance:** Offering empathetic communication to address patient concerns during stressful situations.

> *Example:* An LPN educates a patient recovering from surgery on how to care for their incision and reassures them about the healing process.

2.3.2 Responsibilities Reserved for RNs

While Licensed Practical Nurses (LPNs) are integral to the healthcare team, certain responsibilities are reserved for Registered Nurses (RNs) or other advanced practitioners. These tasks require advanced clinical judgment, critical thinking, and a higher level of training. Recognizing these distinctions ensures that care is delivered safely and within regulatory guidelines, reinforcing the collaborative nature of nursing practice.

Initiating Blood Transfusions

The initiation of blood transfusions is a complex process that requires comprehensive assessment and close monitoring to prevent and address potential complications, such as allergic reactions or hemolysis. This task involves:

- **Pre-Transfusion Assessment:** The RN performs a detailed review of the patient's history, including any previous transfusion reactions, and confirms compatibility between the donor blood and the patient's blood type.
- **Patient Preparation:** Educating the patient about the procedure, including potential side effects and signs of complications, is critical. The RN ensures that informed consent is obtained.

- **Monitoring During Initiation:** The RN monitors the patient closely during the initial 15 minutes, as most adverse reactions occur during this period.

While LPNs are not authorized to initiate transfusions, they play a supporting role by:

- Monitoring vital signs after the transfusion has begun.
- Observing the patient for delayed reactions, such as fever or itching.
- Reporting abnormalities to the RN immediately.

Case Example: An RN initiates a blood transfusion for a patient with anemia, conducting a pre-transfusion assessment and starting the infusion. The LPN assists by checking vital signs every 15 minutes after the transfusion starts and promptly alerts the RN when the patient reports chills, a potential sign of a febrile reaction.

Developing and Modifying Care Plans

RNs are responsible for creating and modifying nursing care plans based on a comprehensive assessment of patient progress and evolving needs. These plans guide the care provided by all team members and ensure that interventions are aligned with the patient's goals and condition.

- **Initial Care Plan Development:** This involves setting priorities, establishing patient-specific goals, and selecting appropriate interventions. For instance, an RN developing a care plan for a patient with heart failure might include interventions to reduce fluid overload and improve oxygenation.
- **Ongoing Adjustments:** As patients' conditions change, the RN evaluates outcomes and revises the plan accordingly.

LPNs contribute to care planning by:

- Reporting observations, such as changes in vital signs or wound healing progress.
- Implementing aspects of the care plan, such as administering medications or providing wound care.

Case Example: An RN revises a care plan for a patient with diabetes after noting persistent high blood glucose levels. The LPN reports that the patient is not adhering to their dietary recommendations, prompting the RN to include dietary counseling as part of the revised plan.

Performing Complex Assessments

Comprehensive assessments require advanced training and are critical for identifying subtle or complex changes in a patient's condition. These assessments often inform significant clinical decisions and are therefore reserved for RNs. Examples include:

- **Neurological Assessments:** Evaluating cranial nerve function, assessing pupil reactivity, and monitoring for signs of increased intracranial pressure are responsibilities of the RN.

- **Interpretation of Diagnostic Results:** RNs analyze lab values, imaging results, and other diagnostics to guide patient care. For example, they might identify trends in electrolyte imbalances that require intervention.

LPNs support these processes by:

- Gathering preliminary data, such as checking pupil reactivity or recording a patient's level of consciousness.
- Reporting findings that indicate a need for further assessment.

> *Case Example:* An RN performs a detailed neurological assessment for a patient with a suspected stroke, including testing for strength, coordination, and reflexes. The LPN assists by documenting the patient's initial responses to verbal stimuli and reporting changes in their level of alertness during their shift.

Administering Complex Treatments

Certain treatments, such as chemotherapy or titrated IV infusions (e.g., heparin drips), are reserved for RNs due to their potential risks and the need for close monitoring.

- RNs administer these treatments after conducting a thorough assessment and ensuring that all safety protocols are in place.
- LPNs may assist by monitoring the patient during treatment and reporting any signs of adverse effects.

> *Case Example:* An RN administers a chemotherapy infusion, checking the patient's labs and ensuring that the dosage aligns with their treatment plan. The LPN observes for immediate side effects, such as nausea or fatigue, and communicates findings to the RN.

2.3.3 Tasks Requiring Collaboration with RNs or Other Team Members

Healthcare delivery often involves collaborative efforts to ensure safe and effective care. LPNs play a pivotal role in teamwork by working closely with RNs and other professionals. Examples of collaborative tasks include:

1. **Wound Care**

   For complex wounds requiring advanced dressings or debridement, LPNs may clean the wound and apply dressings under the direction of a wound care nurse or RN. Collaboration ensures that the treatment plan is followed and adjusted based on the wound's healing progress.

2. **Medication Reconciliation**

   LPNs gather information about a patient's medications during admission or discharge and share this data with the RN or pharmacist for review. This teamwork reduces the risk of medication errors and ensures accuracy in the patient's medication regimen.

3. **Monitoring IV Therapy**

   While LPNs can monitor IV infusions and report findings, they often work with RNs to manage complications or adjust infusion rates based on patient needs.

2.3.4 Legal and Professional Boundaries in Evaluating Orders

Understanding and adhering to legal and professional boundaries is essential for LPNs when accepting assignments or evaluating care orders. Key considerations include:

1. **State Nurse Practice Acts**

   Each state defines the LPN's scope of practice through its nurse practice act. LPNs must be familiar with their state's regulations to ensure compliance. For example, some states allow LPNs to administer IV medications, while others restrict this practice.

2. **Facility Policies**

   Healthcare facilities may have specific policies that further define the LPN's role. For instance, a hospital may permit LPNs to monitor telemetry readings but require RNs to interpret the data and adjust treatment plans.

3. **Refusing Unsafe Assignments**

   If a task exceeds the LPN's training or scope, they must refuse the assignment and escalate the concern to a supervisor. For example, if asked to perform an advanced cardiac assessment, the LPN should explain that this task requires RN expertise and request support.

Examples of Safe and Effective Order Evaluation

1. **Example 1: Medication Administration**

   An LPN receives an order to administer a new antibiotic to a patient with a history of severe penicillin allergy. Recognizing the risk, the LPN verifies the medication with the prescribing provider, ensuring patient safety by avoiding a potential allergic reaction.

2. **Example 2: Delegating Specimen Collection**

   A patient requires a urine culture, but the LPN is occupied with a higher-priority task. The LPN delegates the collection to a trained unlicensed assistive personnel (UAP) and verifies that the sample is collected and labeled properly, maintaining responsibility for the task's outcome.

3. **Example 3: Monitoring Blood Transfusions**

   While an RN initiates a blood transfusion, the LPN monitors the patient's vital signs and observes for adverse reactions, such as fever or hives. If the patient exhibits signs of a reaction, the LPN immediately notifies the RN, ensuring timely intervention.

2.4 Participate in Emergency Preparedness

Licensed Practical Nurses (LPNs) play a vital role in planning, responding to, and managing emergencies, working collaboratively with the healthcare team to mitigate risks and maintain continuity of care. Whether facing natural disasters, fire emergencies, workplace violence, or technological crises, LPNs must be equipped with the knowledge and skills to act decisively.

2.4.1 Identifying and Managing Internal Disasters

Internal disasters are emergencies that originate within a healthcare facility, disrupting operations and endangering patients, staff, and resources. Licensed Practical Nurses (LPNs) are key responders in these situations, tasked with quickly identifying risks, implementing safety measures, and ensuring the continuation of patient care. Internal disasters include utility failures, power outages, workplace violence, and environmental threats such as tornadoes or chemical spills. By adhering to established protocols, LPNs play a pivotal role in minimizing harm and maintaining a safe environment.

Utility Failures and Power Outages

Utility failures and power outages can have serious implications, especially in settings where critical equipment supports patient care. LPNs must act promptly to address these challenges while prioritizing patient safety.

1. **Life-Support Equipment**
    - Patients on ventilators, oxygen therapy, or dialysis machines depend on uninterrupted power supply. LPNs ensure that these devices are connected to backup generators or battery-powered alternatives.
    - For instance, a ventilator-dependent patient in the ICU requires immediate attention during a power outage to avoid respiratory distress. LPNs collaborate with the healthcare team to verify generator functionality and manually assist with ventilation if needed.
2. **Communication and Prioritization**
    - LPNs notify the healthcare team about utility failures and participate in triaging patients based on urgency.
    - For example, in a power outage affecting the operating room, LPNs assist in transferring stable patients to recovery areas while ensuring that critically ill patients receive uninterrupted care.
3. **Monitoring and Documentation**
    - Throughout the outage, LPNs monitor patients for signs of deterioration, such as hypoxia or arrhythmias, and document observations to guide interventions.

- For example, if a patient on oxygen therapy shows signs of respiratory distress, the LPN immediately notifies the RN or physician and provides supplemental oxygen using portable tanks.

Workplace Violence

Workplace violence poses a unique threat in healthcare settings, often arising from agitated patients, visitors, or coworkers. LPNs must be vigilant in identifying warning signs, such as verbal aggression, erratic behavior, or threatening language, and take proactive measures to de-escalate situations.

1. **Recognizing Risks**
   - LPNs observe for potential triggers, such as long wait times, miscommunication, or patients with a history of violent behavior. For example, a patient who becomes increasingly agitated while waiting for test results may exhibit behaviors requiring intervention.
2. **Notifying Security Personnel**
   - Early reporting to security personnel can prevent escalation. For instance, an LPN encountering a visitor shouting at staff notifies security and follows protocol to protect others in the area.
3. **Active Threat Response**
   - During an active threat, such as a physical altercation, LPNs prioritize patient safety by securing doors, moving patients away from danger, and providing reassurance to reduce anxiety.
   - For example, in an incident involving a violent visitor in a clinic, the LPN guides ambulatory patients to a secure room while staying with non-ambulatory patients to ensure their safety.

Environmental Threats

Environmental threats such as tornadoes and chemical spills require immediate action to protect patients and staff from harm. LPNs play a crucial role in implementing safety protocols tailored to each situation.

1. **Tornado Warnings**
   - In the event of a tornado warning, LPNs assist in moving patients to designated safe zones, such as interior hallways or rooms without windows.
   - They ensure patients are positioned safely, using wheelchairs, stretchers, or manual assistance as needed, and provide blankets for additional protection.
   - For example, during a tornado warning, an LPN helps move ICU patients to a central hallway while ensuring portable oxygen tanks and emergency supplies are readily available.

2. **Chemical Spills**

   - Chemical spills require swift action to prevent exposure to hazardous substances. LPNs follow decontamination procedures, such as donning appropriate personal protective equipment (PPE) and assisting affected patients.
   - They ensure contaminated individuals are moved to a designated decontamination area, such as a shower station, and provide support during the process.
   - For instance, if a cleaning agent spill causes respiratory irritation in patients, the LPN relocates them to a well-ventilated area and notifies environmental services for cleanup.

2.4.2 Patient Evacuation Principles

Patient evacuation during emergencies is a highly coordinated process requiring detailed planning and efficient execution to ensure safety while minimizing risks. LPNs are vital participants in evacuation procedures, working collaboratively with the healthcare team to address patient needs while adhering to safety protocols. Evacuations are categorized as **horizontal** or **vertical**, depending on the severity and type of threat. Each type demands specific actions and considerations to ensure patient safety and continuity of care.

Horizontal Evacuations

Horizontal evacuations involve moving patients from one area of a floor to a safer location on the same level. This approach is used when the threat, such as a fire or gas leak, is localized and does not compromise the structural integrity of the facility.

Key Responsibilities for LPNs:

- **Patient Transport:** LPNs assist in transferring patients using wheelchairs, stretchers, or evacuation chairs, ensuring that patients with limited mobility are prioritized.
- **Medication and Records:** Securing essential medications, such as insulin or rescue inhalers, and critical medical records ensures continuity of care after relocation.
- **Clear Communication:** LPNs explain the situation to patients calmly, providing reassurance and instructions to minimize anxiety and ensure cooperation.

> *Example Scenario:* A small fire breaks out in a storage room on a hospital floor. Smoke begins to affect nearby patient rooms, prompting a horizontal evacuation. LPNs assist in moving patients to a smoke-free wing, ensuring that portable oxygen tanks are secured for patients with respiratory needs. They calmly explain the situation to patients and staff, helping to maintain order during the transition.

Vertical Evacuations

Vertical evacuations involve moving patients to a different floor, typically downward, in response to severe threats that render the current floor unsafe, such as major fires, flooding, or structural damage. These evacuations are more complex due to the physical challenges of navigating stairways with patients and equipment.

Key Responsibilities for LPNs:

- **Avoiding Elevators:** Since elevators may become inoperative or unsafe during emergencies, LPNs use stairwells and assist patients with evacuation chairs or stretchers.
- **Team Coordination:** Collaboration with other healthcare providers ensures that patients are prioritized based on their condition, with the most critical patients evacuated first.
- **Patient Safety:** LPNs secure patients during transport, ensuring they remain stable and comfortable while navigating stairways.

Example Scenario: In a multi-story hospital, a significant fire on the upper floors triggers a vertical evacuation. LPNs assist ICU patients by placing them in evacuation chairs and carefully guiding them down the stairwell to a lower floor. Portable monitors and medications are brought along to maintain critical care during the transition.

Critical Considerations

1. **Avoid Using Elevators**

   Elevators may fail or become unsafe during emergencies, especially in cases of power outages or fires. LPNs ensure stairwells are used for evacuation and provide extra support for patients with limited mobility.

2. **Prioritizing Mobility Challenges**

   Patients with mobility impairments, such as those in wheelchairs or requiring assistance to walk, are prioritized during evacuations. LPNs work with the team to ensure these patients receive prompt attention.

3. **Clear Communication with Patients**

   During evacuations, LPNs maintain open lines of communication, explaining the process to patients in simple and reassuring terms. For example:

   > "We're moving to a safer area to keep everyone protected. Stay calm, and we'll guide you step by step."

4. **Ensuring Continuity of Care**

   LPNs ensure critical supplies, such as medications, portable oxygen tanks, and patient records, accompany patients during the evacuation to prevent interruptions in care.

2.4.3 Practical Scenarios Illustrating Disaster Response Protocols

Practical scenarios help illustrate how Licensed Practical Nurses (LPNs) can effectively respond to emergencies, ensuring patient safety and maintaining the continuity of care. These examples highlight the importance of following established protocols and demonstrate the critical role LPNs play in mitigating risks and restoring normal operations.

Fire Emergency

Scenario: A fire breaks out in the hospital kitchen, causing smoke to spread to adjacent areas and triggering the facility's fire alarm. LPNs on a nearby floor act swiftly, following the established RACE protocol:

- **R: Rescue patients in immediate danger**
  LPNs prioritize moving patients closest to the fire or smoke to a safer location. For example, patients in rooms adjacent to the kitchen are immediately evacuated to a smoke-free wing.
- **A: Activate the fire alarm**
  An LPN pulls the nearest fire alarm and notifies the hospital's emergency response team, ensuring that firefighters and facility staff are alerted promptly.
- **C: Confine the fire by closing doors**
  LPNs close doors to patient rooms and other areas to contain the spread of smoke and flames, reducing the risk to other parts of the building.
- **E: Extinguish small fires if trained and safe to do so**
  If the fire is small and manageable, trained LPNs use a fire extinguisher to douse the flames while ensuring their own safety.

Horizontal Evacuation: Patients in the affected wing are evacuated to a safe zone on the same floor. LPNs:

- Use wheelchairs, stretchers, or assist ambulatory patients to move quickly and safely.
- Ensure that portable oxygen tanks and essential medications accompany patients.
- Monitor patients for signs of smoke inhalation, such as coughing, shortness of breath, or disorientation, and report findings to the healthcare team.

Follow-Up Actions: After the immediate threat is contained, LPNs document the incident, including patient locations and any medical concerns that arose during the evacuation. They participate in debriefings to identify improvements for future fire response efforts.

Computer Hacking Episode

Scenario: The hospital's electronic health record (EHR) system is compromised during a hacking incident, disrupting access to critical patient information. LPNs adapt quickly to maintain patient care while safeguarding sensitive data.

Switch to Paper Documentation:

- LPNs revert to using paper documentation to record essential information such as medication schedules, vital signs, and care notes.
- They ensure accuracy and legibility in their entries to facilitate smooth transitions when the EHR system is restored.

Securing Patient Information:

- Sensitive data is protected by locking paper records in secure storage areas when not in use.
- LPNs avoid discussing patient information in public spaces, reducing the risk of breaches.

Coordination with IT and Leadership:

- LPNs report system issues promptly to the IT department and follow their guidance to avoid further compromise.
- They communicate effectively with team members to share updates and ensure all staff are informed of temporary documentation processes.

Example Response: A patient with diabetes requires insulin during the hacking incident. The LPN verifies the dose from the most recent printed medical record, administers the insulin, and documents the action manually. The LPN ensures that the paper documentation is stored securely and updates the RN and care team about the patient's current status.

2.5 Ensure Safe Client Handling

Ensuring safe client handling is a fundamental responsibility of Licensed Practical Nurses (LPNs) to protect both patients and caregivers from injury during routine care, emergencies, and preoperative preparations. Proper application of body mechanics, safe handling techniques, and attention to detail are critical in minimizing risks and enhancing patient outcomes. From routine repositioning to managing preoperative preparation and handling urgent care scenarios, LPNs play a pivotal role in maintaining safety and comfort.

2.5.1 Applying Proper Body Mechanics and Safe Handling Techniques

Proper body mechanics and safe handling techniques are essential for preventing injuries in caregivers and ensuring patient safety during routine transfers and repositioning. Licensed Practical Nurses (LPNs) play a critical role in implementing these practices, which not only protect their own physical health but also contribute to the patient's comfort and well-being. Mastering these techniques reduces the risk of falls, musculoskeletal injuries, and other complications during patient care.

A stable base is the foundation of safe lifting and handling.

- **Foot Position:** LPNs should stand with feet shoulder-width apart and one foot slightly forward to distribute weight evenly and enhance balance. This stance reduces the risk of losing footing, especially when handling heavy or unpredictable movements.

- **Postural Alignment:** Keep the spine in a neutral position, avoiding excessive arching or rounding of the back. Proper alignment minimizes strain on the lower back and core muscles.

> *Example:* When repositioning a patient in bed, the LPN adjusts their feet to maintain a stable base, ensuring they can shift weight efficiently without twisting their spine.

Using the leg muscles, rather than the back, is a cornerstone of proper lifting techniques.

- **Knee Bending:** Bend at the knees while keeping the back straight, allowing the stronger leg muscles to bear the weight.
- **Avoid Overreaching:** Keep the load close to the body to minimize leverage that could strain the lower back.

> *Example:* When assisting a patient from a chair to a standing position, the LPN bends their knees, supports the patient's arms or gait belt, and avoids bending forward at the waist, which could result in back injuries.

Assistive devices reduce physical strain and improve the safety of patient transfers, particularly for patients with limited mobility.

- **Gait Belts:** These belts provide a secure grip for caregivers to support patients during transfers or ambulation. LPNs ensure the belt is snug but not restrictive, positioned around the patient's waist.
- **Transfer Boards:** These boards allow smooth lateral transfers, such as moving a patient from a wheelchair to a bed. LPNs ensure the surfaces are level and instruct the patient to shift gradually with assistance.
- **Mechanical Lifts:** These are essential for moving non-ambulatory patients. LPNs ensure the sling is positioned correctly, check weight limits, and operate the lift steadily to prevent discomfort or injury.

> *Example:* During a routine transfer of a patient with limited mobility from a bed to a wheelchair, an LPN utilizes a gait belt to assist the patient. They position the wheelchair at a 45-degree angle to the bed and lock its brakes to ensure stability. The LPN instructs the patient to place their hands on the armrests for support, bends at the knees to maintain proper body mechanics, and uses the gait belt to guide the patient into the wheelchair safely.

2.5.2 Preoperative Preparation and Hazard Prevention

Preoperative preparation involves addressing potential hazards to ensure patient safety during surgery. LPNs play an essential role in identifying and mitigating risks, such as:

- **Removing Personal Belongings:** Items such as jewelry, contact lenses, and dentures must be removed to prevent complications during surgery. For example, contact lenses can cause corneal drying if left in place, while jewelry may interfere with electrical equipment or pose a choking hazard.

- **Documentation and Storage:** Personal belongings should be labeled and stored securely to prevent loss.

Practical Example: Before surgery, an LPN assists a patient by removing contact lenses and storing them in a labeled case. The LPN also ensures that the patient's jewelry is placed in a secure bag and documented in the patient's chart.

- **Comfort and Safety:** LPNs help alleviate preoperative anxiety by explaining procedures, addressing patient concerns, and ensuring physical comfort.

Preventing Complications: LPNs monitor for potential issues, such as ensuring the patient's eyes are closed and covered with protective ointment or shields to prevent corneal drying during general anesthesia.

2.5.3 Safe Transfers During Emergencies

In emergency situations, the ability to perform safe and efficient patient transfers is critical to ensuring the well-being of both patients and caregivers. Licensed Practical Nurses (LPNs) must adapt quickly to dynamic scenarios, using appropriate techniques and equipment to minimize risks while maintaining a calm and organized approach. Emergencies such as fires, natural disasters, or structural damage may require immediate action, and LPNs play a vital role in these high-pressure situations.

Using Emergency Techniques

When patients are non-ambulatory or unable to assist in their evacuation, LPNs employ specialized emergency transfer methods:

- **Evacuation Chairs:** Designed for stairway use, evacuation chairs allow LPNs to safely transport non-ambulatory patients during emergencies such as fires. These chairs are particularly useful in multi-story facilities where elevators are inaccessible.
- **Stretchers:** For patients requiring horizontal positioning, stretchers provide a secure means of transfer. LPNs ensure that the patient is properly strapped to the stretcher to prevent slipping during movement.
- **Improvised Techniques:** In resource-limited situations, LPNs may need to use blanket drags or manual carries to move patients. For example, a blanket drag involves placing the patient on a sturdy blanket and carefully pulling them to safety, ensuring that their head and neck are supported.

Example: During a fire evacuation in a hospital, an LPN uses an evacuation chair to transport a non-ambulatory patient down a flight of stairs. The LPN collaborates with another team member to secure the patient's portable oxygen tank and monitors the patient for signs of distress throughout the transfer.

Minimizing Risk of Injury

In emergency transfers, preventing further harm to the patient is a top priority. LPNs must ensure that the patient's body remains properly aligned during movement to reduce the risk of fractures, spinal injuries, or dislocations.

- **Proper Body Alignment:** LPNs check that the patient's head, neck, and spine are aligned before initiating any transfer. If a spinal injury is suspected, the patient is moved using a spinal board or log roll technique to maintain alignment.
- **Controlled Movements:** Sudden or jerky movements are avoided to minimize discomfort and the risk of injury. For example, when using a blanket drag, the LPN pulls steadily and avoids sharp tugs.
- **Supportive Positioning:** Non-ambulatory patients are secured with straps or padding to prevent shifting during movement.

Example: During an earthquake evacuation, an LPN assists a patient with a suspected pelvic fracture. The LPN ensures the patient is stabilized on a stretcher with proper padding to immobilize the pelvis and coordinates with the team to move the stretcher safely to an outdoor triage area.

Team Coordination and Communication

Safe transfers during emergencies often require collaboration with other healthcare team members. Clear communication and role assignments are crucial to ensuring smooth and efficient evacuations.

- **Assigning Roles:** LPNs may delegate specific tasks, such as managing medical equipment or guiding ambulatory patients, to other team members.
- **Maintaining Communication:** LPNs keep patients informed about what to expect during the transfer, which helps reduce anxiety and fosters cooperation. For example, an LPN might reassure a patient during a fire evacuation by explaining, "We're taking you to a safe area now. Please hold onto the armrests, and we'll guide you step by step."
- **Coordinating Equipment Use:** During emergencies, LPNs ensure that evacuation equipment such as stretchers, oxygen tanks, and portable monitors are readily available and properly used.

Example: In a hurricane evacuation scenario, an LPN leads a team to transfer ICU patients to a safer floor. The LPN assigns roles for managing ventilators and securing intravenous lines, ensuring that critical care equipment is transported with the patient.

2.6 Identify and Address Unsafe Conditions

Recognizing and addressing unsafe conditions in healthcare settings is fundamental to protecting clients, staff, and the overall integrity of care. LPNs play a pivotal role in identifying hazards, taking prompt action, and escalating concerns when necessary. By maintaining vigilance, adhering to legal and ethical responsibilities, and fostering a culture of accountability, LPNs contribute significantly to a safe and respectful healthcare environment.

LPNs must continuously monitor the healthcare environment for safety risks that could compromise patient care or staff well-being. These hazards can include:

- **Discrepancies in Narcotic Counts:** Inconsistent narcotic inventory may indicate medication errors, theft, or misuse. LPNs should document any discrepancies and report them to the charge nurse or pharmacy immediately. Escalation to the state Board of Nursing may be required for unresolved or serious issues.
- **Abuse or Neglect:** Suspicion of physical, emotional, or verbal abuse toward clients must be addressed immediately. For example, signs of neglect such as malnutrition, poor hygiene, or unexplained injuries should prompt LPNs to notify the appropriate authorities or mandated reporters within the institution.
- **Inappropriate Conduct:** Verbal or physical assault within the healthcare team undermines client safety and must be reported to supervisors or human resources.

Scenario: An LPN observes a colleague verbally berating a client in distress. The LPN documents the incident and reports it to the charge nurse, following institutional policies for addressing inappropriate behavior.

2.6.1 Addressing Client-Specific Safety Risks

Certain client conditions require heightened vigilance to ensure safety and prevent complications, particularly when dealing with postoperative clients or those with complex medical needs. Post-transsphenoidal surgery patients, for instance, are at increased risk for airway compromise due to nasal congestion or swelling. In such cases, LPNs play a crucial role in closely monitoring for signs of respiratory distress, such as labored breathing, decreased oxygen saturation, or cyanosis. Any indications of difficulty should prompt immediate action, including notifying the care team and implementing appropriate interventions. For example, providing humidified oxygen can help alleviate dryness and congestion, while suctioning may be necessary to maintain a patent airway. Elevating the head of the bed to reduce pressure and facilitate breathing is another effective strategy. Prompt communication with the RN or provider ensures that emergent issues are addressed without delay.

The early recognition of complications extends beyond respiratory concerns. LPNs must remain alert to subtle changes in a patient's condition, such as abnormal vital signs, altered mental status, or unexpected pain, which can indicate underlying issues. A client recovering from transsphenoidal surgery, for example, may report increasing difficulty breathing due to nasal obstruction. In response, the LPN elevates the head of the bed, administers humidified oxygen, and promptly informs the RN to initiate further evaluation by the provider. These actions demonstrate the importance of timely intervention in mitigating potential complications and ensuring the patient's safety and comfort.

When safety risks are identified, LPNs must know how to escalate concerns effectively to ensure proper resolution. Reporting to the charge nurse or supervisor is often the first step in addressing hazards, whether related to improper medication administration, unsafe patient handling, or environmental dangers. For more significant issues, such as suspected abuse or systemic safety failures, LPNs may need to escalate the matter further by involving appropriate authorities, such as the state Board of Nursing, risk management, or even law enforcement. In such cases, clear documentation and adherence to established reporting protocols are essential for ensuring transparency and accountability.

Legal and ethical considerations also play a critical role in addressing client-specific safety risks. As mandated reporters, nurses are legally required to report suspicions of abuse or neglect, even in the absence of certainty. This obligation ensures that investigations can occur to protect vulnerable individuals and uphold ethical standards within the healthcare environment. For example, an LPN who identifies a discrepancy in narcotic counts during the end-of-shift inventory must act decisively to address the issue. After verifying the records, the LPN reports the discrepancy to the charge nurse and documents the findings accurately and thoroughly. This action not only resolves an immediate safety concern but also upholds the integrity of the healthcare team and reinforces a culture of accountability.

2.6.2 Addressing Unsafe Conditions for Staff

Protecting staff requires a proactive approach to identifying and mitigating risks, ensuring a safe and secure working environment for everyone. One key area of concern is radiation exposure, particularly for staff working with radioactive clients or equipment. LPNs must be familiar with institutional policies and adhere to radiation safety guidelines to minimize exposure. This includes using personal protective equipment (PPE), such as lead aprons or shields, and ensuring proper signage and restricted access to areas where radioactive materials are in use. Vulnerable staff members, such as pregnant nurses, require special consideration. Assignments involving radioactive materials should be avoided whenever possible to protect both the nurse and the developing fetus. If such an assignment is made inadvertently, the LPN has a responsibility to advocate for the nurse by ensuring that the task is reassigned in compliance with safety protocols. For example, an LPN might delegate care for a client undergoing radiation therapy to another team member, prioritizing the health and safety of the pregnant nurse while maintaining continuity of care.

Workplace safety also encompasses a wide range of other hazards, from malfunctioning equipment to environmental risks like wet floors or cluttered evacuation routes. LPNs must be vigilant in identifying these issues and addressing them promptly to prevent accidents or injuries. Malfunctioning equipment, for instance, should be reported to maintenance staff immediately, and faulty items should be removed from service to avoid potential harm. Clear evacuation routes are essential for emergency preparedness, and LPNs should ensure that hallways and exits remain free of obstructions. Environmental hazards like wet floors or improperly stored items should be addressed without delay to reduce the risk of slips, trips, and falls.

Scenario-driven interventions further highlight the importance of addressing unsafe conditions for staff. For example, if a pregnant nurse is inadvertently assigned to care for a client undergoing radiation therapy, the LPN steps in to ensure that the task is reassigned in compliance with institutional policies. This involves clear communication with supervisors and collaboration with the team to balance workload distribution while upholding safety standards. Similarly, if an LPN encounters a piece of malfunctioning equipment, they promptly remove it from use, report the issue to the appropriate department, and document the action to ensure accountability.

Task Delegation and Assignment Strategies

Delegation and task assignment play an integral role in fostering a safe healthcare environment:

- **Prioritizing Safety:** Assign tasks based on staff competencies and avoid delegating responsibilities beyond an individual's training or scope of practice.
- **Compliance with Standards:** Ensure all team members understand institutional policies and adhere to safety protocols, such as proper infection control measures or medication administration procedures.

Scenario: An LPN delegates vital sign monitoring for a stable client to a trained unlicensed assistive personnel (UAP) but retains responsibility for interpreting the results and addressing any abnormalities. This approach maintains safety while promoting efficiency.

Proactive Risk Identification and Intervention

A proactive approach to safety involves constant vigilance and accountability:

- **Routine Inspections:** LPNs regularly inspect the care environment for hazards, such as exposed electrical wires or improperly stored medications, and take immediate action to address them.
- **Education and Advocacy:** LPNs educate staff and clients about potential risks, such as fall prevention measures or proper handling of sharps, and advocate for necessary changes to improve safety.

Scenario: An LPN notices a spill in a hallway that poses a slipping hazard. The LPN places a caution sign at the site, informs housekeeping staff, and ensures the area is cleaned promptly.

Examples of Unsafe Conditions and Responses

1. **Improper Handling of Radioactive Clients**
    - *Unsafe Condition:* A client undergoing radiation therapy is placed in a shared room without consideration for radiation exposure limits.
    - *Response:* The LPN notifies the charge nurse, relocates the client to an appropriate room, and ensures signage is placed to warn staff and visitors of radiation precautions.

2. **Suspected Abuse**
   - *Unsafe Condition:* A pediatric client exhibits unexplained bruises and avoids eye contact with caregivers.
   - *Response:* The LPN reports the observations to the supervisor and documents the findings, initiating the mandated reporting process to protect the child.
3. **Discrepancies in Care Practices**
   - *Unsafe Condition:* A colleague skips hand hygiene before performing a wound dressing change.
   - *Response:* The LPN addresses the issue directly with the colleague, reinforces infection control protocols, and reports the incident if the behavior persists.

2.7 Follow Timed Monitoring Protocols

LPNs must regularly assess and monitor clients based on established schedules, the urgency of their conditions, and standard procedural timelines. Effective prioritization and timely intervention are particularly critical when caring for clients with high-risk conditions or managing multiple clients in settings like home health. By recognizing the specific needs of each client and implementing a structured approach to monitoring, LPNs can optimize outcomes and maintain safety.

Regular monitoring requires vigilance and adherence to established schedules for routine assessments and procedures. For example, postoperative suture or staple removal is typically performed according to a standard timeline based on the surgeon's recommendations and the client's healing progress. Before proceeding, LPNs must evaluate the site for signs of readiness, such as the absence of swelling, redness, or drainage, and ensure that the client has received appropriate follow-up care instructions. Careful assessment of the healing process minimizes the risk of complications such as infection or delayed wound closure.

In high-risk clients, the need for frequent and timely monitoring becomes even more urgent. Conditions such as airway or breathing issues, central lines, severe infections, or complex treatment regimens necessitate immediate evaluation and intervention when complications arise. For instance, a client with congestive heart failure (CHF) who experiences nighttime dyspnea requires prompt assessment to prevent respiratory distress. Similarly, clients with potential airway alterations, such as those with laryngeal cancer or a recent laryngectomy, must be monitored closely for signs of airway compromise, including stridor, difficulty swallowing, or changes in oxygen saturation. Early recognition and intervention in these cases are vital for preventing life-threatening outcomes.

In home health settings, where nurses may care for multiple clients with varying levels of acuity, prioritizing care is crucial. LPNs must evaluate each client's condition to determine who requires immediate attention and who can be seen later in the schedule. For example, a client with a central line at risk for infection or thrombosis takes precedence over a stable client with routine medication management needs. Strategies for effective prioritization include organizing visits geographically, clustering clients with similar care needs, and allowing flexibility to accommodate urgent situations.

Timely intervention and scheduling efficiency are also key components of effective monitoring. LPNs must identify and prioritize life-threatening conditions, such as airway or breathing concerns, over less urgent needs. This requires making informed decisions based on clinical judgment, client history, and current symptoms. For example, a client recovering from a laryngectomy who exhibits difficulty breathing and cyanosis should be evaluated and treated immediately, even if it means rescheduling a routine visit for another client. Addressing urgent concerns first ensures that critical needs are met without compromising overall care quality.

Effective planning is an essential skill for LPNs tasked with managing multiple clients. By assessing each client's acuity and risk level, LPNs can create a structured visit schedule that minimizes complications and improves outcomes. High-risk clients, such as those with severe infections or complex treatment regimens, are prioritized to ensure they receive timely and appropriate care. For example, an LPN providing home care may schedule a morning visit for a client with a fever and a suspected bloodstream infection to initiate antibiotic therapy promptly, while deferring a routine wellness check for a stable client to later in the day.

Scenarios further illustrate the importance of prioritization and adherence to monitoring protocols. In a hospital setting, an LPN may be responsible for monitoring several postoperative clients. If one client reports increasing pain and swelling around a surgical site, the LPN evaluates the area immediately for signs of infection, such as warmth, redness, or drainage, and informs the RN or provider to initiate treatment. Meanwhile, other clients who are stable continue to receive care according to their monitoring schedules. In home health, an LPN managing a client with CHF who has experienced worsening shortness of breath prioritizes this visit over a routine medication review, ensuring timely intervention and reducing the risk of hospitalization.

2.8 Provide and Maintain Safety Equipment

LPNs are responsible for verifying that essential medical devices are functional, accessible, and correctly maintained. This involves adhering to maintenance protocols, educating clients on safe equipment use, and ensuring readiness to address urgent needs. By emphasizing proper equipment handling and client education, LPNs play a crucial role in fostering a safe healthcare environment.

Ensuring that specialized tools are available and in good working order is a critical aspect of maintaining safety equipment. For example, in cases involving crutchfield tongs—a device used for cervical spine stabilization—a torque wrench must be readily available to adjust the tongs as needed. This ensures proper alignment and prevents device-related complications, such as insufficient traction or damage to the cervical spine. LPNs should routinely inspect these tools, verify their functionality, and ensure they are accessible at the bedside for emergencies. Additionally, maintaining proper documentation of equipment checks and addressing issues immediately reinforces the reliability of safety equipment.

In urgent situations, having the appropriate equipment at the bedside can make the difference between a successful intervention and a critical delay. Examples include maintaining functional oxygen delivery systems, suction devices, or defibrillators to manage airway or cardiac emergencies. LPNs are responsible for performing regular equipment checks, such as ensuring oxygen tanks are full and suction devices are properly assembled. For instance, a patient recovering from surgery who suddenly develops respiratory distress requires immediate access to a functioning suction device to clear the airway and prevent further complications.

Proper handling and maintenance protocols are essential for preventing equipment failure and ensuring readiness for use. LPNs must follow institutional guidelines for cleaning, storing, and servicing medical devices. For example, reusable equipment like crutchfield tongs or infusion pumps should be cleaned and inspected between uses to ensure they remain sterile and functional. LPNs should also collaborate with the biomedical team to report and address malfunctioning devices promptly, minimizing risks to client safety.

In addition to maintaining equipment, LPNs are instrumental in educating clients on the safe use and management of medical devices, such as implantable defibrillators. These devices, which regulate heart rhythms, require careful handling to prevent malfunctions or interference. Clients should be advised to keep electronic devices, such as cellphones, at least six inches away from the defibrillator to avoid electromagnetic interference. Similarly, battery-operated machinery should be used with caution, and clients should be educated on recognizing interference-related symptoms, such as dizziness or fainting. These precautions are critical for ensuring the proper function of the device and avoiding potentially life-threatening complications.

Discharge education is equally important for clients managing medical devices at home. LPNs should provide clear, written instructions on device safety and maintenance, as well as symptoms that warrant immediate medical attention. For example, a client with an implantable defibrillator experiencing frequent shocks, chest pain, or syncope should seek prompt medical evaluation. LPNs should also emphasize the importance of attending regular follow-up appointments to monitor device function and make necessary adjustments.

Practical scenarios highlight the importance of equipment availability, maintenance, and client education in promoting safety. For instance, an LPN caring for a client with crutchfield tongs routinely checks the torque wrench's availability and ensures the tongs are properly aligned. The LPN collaborates with the care team to monitor the client's condition and prevent complications like skin breakdown or infection at the pin sites. Similarly, an LPN providing discharge education to a client with an implantable defibrillator explains the importance of avoiding proximity to electromagnetic fields, outlines safety precautions, and ensures the client understands how to recognize warning signs of device malfunction.

2.9 Implement the Least Restrictive Restraints

The use of restraints, including physical restraints and seclusion, is a highly sensitive area in healthcare that must prioritize client safety and dignity while adhering to strict legal, ethical, and procedural guidelines. Restraints should only be implemented when absolutely necessary to prevent harm to the client or others and after all less restrictive alternatives have been exhausted. LPNs play a vital role in supporting the proper implementation, documentation, and monitoring of restraint use, ensuring compliance with institutional policies and safeguarding client rights.

The decision to use restraints or seclusion must be guided by clear and comprehensive protocols. Seclusion, in particular, involves isolating a client in a controlled environment to prevent harm and requires a qualified professional, such as an RN or physician, to authorize its use. LPNs are responsible for assisting in the process by ensuring that the intervention aligns with established policies and that all alternatives have been considered. For example, a client exhibiting aggressive behavior due to a psychiatric condition may first be approached using de-escalation techniques, such as calm verbal communication or redirection, before seclusion is considered.

When restraints are deemed necessary, LPNs must ensure that the least restrictive option is used to achieve the desired safety outcome. This approach minimizes the impact on the client's mobility and autonomy while effectively addressing the immediate risk. For instance, a client at risk of self-harm might require mittens to prevent them from pulling at an IV line rather than full physical restraints. In cases where seclusion is necessary, LPNs assist in preparing the environment to ensure safety, such as removing potentially harmful objects and providing supervision to monitor the client's well-being.

Monitoring and documentation are critical components of restraint use to ensure compliance with legal and regulatory standards. LPNs must perform frequent checks on restrained clients to assess their physical and emotional status, addressing any discomfort or complications that may arise. For example, a client in wrist restraints should be monitored for signs of impaired circulation, such as discoloration or swelling, and adjustments should be made immediately if issues are identified. Regular repositioning and offering opportunities for hydration, nutrition, and toileting further reinforce the commitment to maintaining client dignity and comfort.

Proper documentation provides accountability and transparency in the use of restraints and seclusion. LPNs record the rationale for the intervention, the alternatives tried, and the client's response before and during its implementation. For seclusion, documentation should include the time the intervention began, the client's behavior, ongoing monitoring observations, and the time seclusion was discontinued. This level of detail ensures that the intervention can be reviewed and evaluated for appropriateness and compliance.

Scenario-based examples illustrate the appropriate use of restraints and seclusion. In one scenario, a client recovering from surgery repeatedly attempts to remove their nasogastric tube, risking complications. After less restrictive measures, such as verbal redirection and distraction, fail, the LPN applies mittens to prevent the client from pulling at the tube. The LPN monitors the client's skin integrity under the mittens and documents the intervention, including its necessity and the client's response. In another scenario, a client with a severe psychiatric condition becomes violent and poses a threat to others in a hospital unit. Following unsuccessful de-escalation attempts, the RN authorizes seclusion. The LPN assists in preparing the seclusion room, removes potentially dangerous objects, and monitors the client continuously, documenting their behavior and any interventions provided.

2.10 Acknowledge and Document Practice Errors

Acknowledging and documenting practice errors is a critical aspect of maintaining client safety, ensuring professional accountability, and fostering a culture of continuous improvement in healthcare. Errors can occur even in the most diligent practices, and LPNs play a vital role in identifying, addressing, and reporting these incidents promptly. Through accurate documentation and adherence to legal, ethical, and professional standards, LPNs contribute to safeguarding patient rights and improving care quality.

When an error is identified, immediate action is necessary to minimize harm and address potential risks. For example, if an LPN discovers a discrepancy in a narcotic count during shift change, the nursing supervisor must be notified immediately, and the chain of command must be followed. This ensures the issue is addressed transparently and prevents further errors. Accurate documentation is critical in such cases, as it establishes a factual account of the incident, protects the integrity of the care team, and provides a foundation for analyzing the root cause of the error.

Errors must be handled in compliance with legal and ethical standards, such as those outlined by the Health Insurance Portability and Accountability Act (HIPAA). Maintaining client confidentiality during the reporting process is essential, and records should only include relevant clinical information. For instance, when documenting a medication administration error, the report should detail the medication given, the dosage, the intended medication, and any immediate interventions provided. Avoid including unnecessary patient identifiers or subjective commentary, as this could compromise the report's professionalism and objectivity.

The process of handling errors involves several key steps. First, the LPN must acknowledge the error and assess the client's condition to determine if any harm has occurred. Timely interventions, such as administering an antidote or notifying the provider, may be necessary to mitigate adverse effects. Next, the LPN must document the incident accurately in both the client's medical record and the facility's incident reporting system. This documentation should include a clear description of the error, the actions taken, and the client's response. For example, if a medication error resulted in an unintended dose of insulin, the LPN would document the administration, the client's blood glucose level, and any corrective measures taken, such as providing glucose or monitoring for hypoglycemia.

Filing a formal incident report is another essential step. Incident reports provide a structured framework for analyzing errors and implementing preventive measures. LPNs should include details such as the time and location of the incident, contributing factors, and recommendations for avoiding similar errors in the future. These reports are reviewed by supervisors and risk management teams to identify patterns, address systemic issues, and promote a safer care environment.

The role of the charge nurse is integral in managing practice errors. Charge nurses oversee the initial response to errors, ensure appropriate documentation, and coordinate follow-up actions. Progressive management strategies may include issuing formal reprimands for repeated errors or escalating concerns to higher authorities if the behavior persists or results in harm. For instance, if an LPN repeatedly fails to follow medication administration protocols despite additional training, the charge nurse may recommend further corrective actions, such as additional education or reassignment.

Creating a culture of accountability and continuous improvement is essential for preventing future errors. LPNs should engage in reflective practice to understand the root causes of mistakes and identify strategies for improvement. Team debriefings and educational sessions can also foster a collaborative approach to learning from errors. For example, a discussion about a near-miss involving medication administration might lead to the implementation of a double-check system to enhance accuracy.

Timely reporting and documentation of errors are vital for maintaining safety standards and protecting patient rights. By acting promptly and transparently, LPNs contribute to an ethical and professional care environment that prioritizes safety and quality. Additionally, compliance with federal laws and institutional policies reinforces the trust and confidence of clients, families, and the healthcare team.

Chapter 3

Health Promotion and Maintenance

This chapter focuses on strategies for disease prevention, fostering healthy behaviors, and guiding clients through developmental milestones. Whether educating clients about nutrition, conducting routine screenings, or addressing life transitions, nurses play a vital role in empowering individuals to take charge of their well-being. By understanding these principles, nurses can contribute to healthier outcomes and a better quality of life for their clients.

3.1 Maternal and Newborn Care

Caring for pregnant clients and newborns requires a strong foundation in both prenatal and postnatal practices. In this section, you will explore essential concepts that guide maternal and newborn nursing—ranging from estimating delivery dates and understanding multifetal pregnancies to supporting labor, postpartum recovery, and the safe care of newborns. You will also review strategies for client education, preventive measures, and coordinated care with other healthcare professionals. By mastering these core principles, you will be better prepared to deliver comprehensive, compassionate care to mothers and their infants.

3.1.1 Prenatal Education and Assessment

Effective prenatal education begins with helping clients understand the importance of accurately estimating the **Estimated Date of Delivery (EDD)**. Knowing the EDD provides a foundation for monitoring the pregnancy, scheduling critical prenatal care milestones, and preparing for labor and delivery.

Calculating EDD Using Nagele's Rule

One of the most widely used methods for estimating the due date is **Nagele's Rule**. This simple formula calculates the EDD by taking the **first day of the client's last menstrual period (LMP)**, subtracting three months, and then adding seven days. For instance:

- If the client's LMP was **April 15th**, subtract three months to get **January 15th**, then add seven days to arrive at an EDD of **January 22nd**.

Providing clients with clear examples and practice problems allows them to become familiar with this method. Encourage them to calculate the EDD for various LMP dates to reinforce the concept and build confidence.

It is crucial to emphasize that the EDD calculated using Nagele's Rule is an estimate and serves as a guideline rather than a fixed date. Only about **5% of pregnancies result in delivery on the exact due date**, with most occurring within two weeks before or after. Clients should understand this variability to avoid unnecessary anxiety.

Other Methods for Determining EDD

In addition to Nagele's Rule, there are other valuable tools for confirming and refining the estimated due date, ensuring that the timeline of the pregnancy is as accurate as possible. One of the most reliable methods is ultrasound imaging, particularly in the first trimester. During this early stage, measurements such as the crown-rump length (CRL) are used to provide precise data about the fetus's development. This information allows healthcare providers to validate or adjust the estimated date of delivery based on objective observations. Ultrasounds also play a crucial role in monitoring the pregnancy's progress, offering reassurance to clients and enabling the early detection of potential complications. When discussing ultrasounds with clients, it is essential to explain how they work and why they are an important part of prenatal care.

Another essential method for determining the EDD involves accurate tracking of menstrual cycles. Encouraging clients to maintain detailed records of their cycles is invaluable. This includes noting the first day of each period, calculating the average length of their cycles, and identifying any irregularities. These details provide crucial context for healthcare providers, allowing them to make informed decisions when calculating gestational age. By supporting clients in developing this habit, they gain a clearer understanding of their reproductive health, which can enhance the accuracy of pregnancy dating and foster greater engagement in their prenatal care.

Relating EDD to Prenatal Milestones

Educating clients about the relationship between the estimated date of delivery (EDD) and the key milestones of pregnancy is essential for fostering a deeper understanding of its progression. Each trimester brings unique changes and challenges, and helping clients grasp these stages allows them to feel more prepared and engaged in their prenatal care journey.

The first trimester, which spans from weeks 1 to 12, is a critical period of development when the foundations for all major organs are established. It is also the time for important early screenings and tests that assess both maternal and fetal health. Clients often find this stage both exciting and overwhelming, so providing clear information about what to expect can help ease their concerns.

During the second trimester, from weeks 13 to 26, the pace of growth accelerates, and many clients will begin to feel fetal movements for the first time—a moment that often strengthens the bond between parent and baby. This trimester also includes anatomy scans, which offer detailed insights into the baby's development and can reassure clients about their progress.

The third trimester, encompassing weeks 27 to 40, is a time of final preparations. Clients can expect significant fetal weight gain and should focus on planning for labor and delivery. Monitoring becomes particularly important during this period to identify and manage any complications that may arise.

By understanding these stages, clients can better anticipate necessary tests, make informed lifestyle adjustments, and schedule healthcare visits effectively. This knowledge equips them to take an active role in their pregnancy and approach each phase with confidence and clarity.

Supporting Clients in Pregnancy Education

Empowering clients to track their pregnancy and understand its progression involves providing them with practical tools and strategies to stay informed and engaged. One effective approach is encouraging the use of a pregnancy calendar or mobile app to monitor key milestones. These tools can help clients visualize their baby's development and plan for upcoming appointments and tests.

Another valuable strategy is guiding clients to keep a journal. By recording symptoms, fetal movements, and any questions they might have for their healthcare provider, clients can stay attuned to their own experiences and communicate more effectively during prenatal visits. Regularly scheduling these visits not only ensures optimal maternal and fetal health but also provides an opportunity for clients to discuss any concerns and receive personalized care.

In addition to these tracking methods, teaching clients about fetal development can deepen their sense of connection to the pregnancy. For example, explaining how the baby's heart begins to beat around six weeks or highlighting the significant weight gain that occurs during the final trimester can make the journey feel more tangible and meaningful. This combination of practical guidance and educational support fosters active participation and helps clients approach their pregnancy with confidence and a stronger emotional bond with their baby.

3.1.2 Support for Laboring Clients

Supporting laboring clients requires a multifaceted approach that includes monitoring the progression of labor, managing discomfort, and ensuring safe and timely interventions. Labor is a dynamic process, and clients benefit from both physical care and emotional reassurance throughout this transformative experience.

Observing Labor Progression and Collaborating in Care

Observing and monitoring labor progression is a critical responsibility for healthcare providers, ensuring the safety of both the client and the newborn. This involves assessing several key indicators, including cervical dilation, effacement, fetal station, and uterine contractions, to determine whether labor is advancing as expected. Cervical dilation measures the opening of the cervix, from 0 centimeters (completely closed) to 10 centimeters (fully dilated), while effacement refers to the thinning and shortening of the cervix, expressed as a percentage. Both must progress adequately for a vaginal delivery to occur. Regular assessments help identify any delays or complications that may require intervention.

Fetal station is another essential parameter, indicating the position of the baby's head in relation to the maternal ischial spines, which are bony landmarks within the pelvis. This measurement, recorded on a scale from -3 (above the ischial spines) to +3 (below the spines and ready for delivery), provides critical information about the baby's descent through the birth canal. A lack of progression in fetal station may suggest potential complications, such as cephalopelvic disproportion, which could necessitate alternative delivery methods like a cesarean section.

Uterine contractions are closely monitored for their frequency, duration, intensity, and resting tone. Effective contractions are key to advancing labor, typically occurring every 2–3 minutes and lasting 60–90 seconds during active labor. Deviations, such as ineffective contractions or uterine hyperstimulation, can pose risks to both mother and baby. These issues may require medical management, including adjustments to medications like oxytocin, to ensure safe and effective labor progression.

When labor does not proceed as expected, prompt recognition of deviations is essential. Prolonged labor can lead to maternal exhaustion, increased infection risk, and fetal distress. Signs of fetal distress, such as abnormal heart rate patterns or meconium-stained amniotic fluid, require immediate attention. Interventions may include repositioning the client, administering oxygen, or preparing for emergency delivery to protect the health of both the mother and the baby.

Effective collaboration among healthcare providers is vital during labor. Licensed practical nurses (LPNs) play an essential role in observing the client, documenting findings, and communicating any changes to the healthcare team. This coordination ensures timely decision-making and intervention. In high-stakes scenarios, such as an emergency cesarean section, clear communication between team members is crucial for managing the situation efficiently and minimizing risks. Teamwork not only ensures the client and newborn's safety but also builds trust and confidence in the care being provided.

Alongside clinical monitoring, emotional and physical support are integral to the care of laboring clients. Providing reassurance, offering pain relief options, assisting with position changes, and encouraging relaxation techniques can significantly enhance the client's comfort and contribute to a positive birthing experience. Empowering clients to participate actively in their care fosters a sense of control and confidence during this transformative process.

Managing Common Pregnancy-Related Discomforts

Managing the physical discomforts that often accompany pregnancy is an essential aspect of providing comprehensive care to clients. Constipation, for example, is a common concern due to hormonal changes and the pressure of the growing uterus on the intestines. Educating clients about simple dietary adjustments can make a significant difference. Increasing fiber intake through fruits, vegetables, and whole grains is a natural way to promote bowel regularity. Additionally, maintaining adequate hydration and incorporating light physical activity, such as walking, are effective strategies for alleviating constipation. Clients should also be cautioned about the use of over-the-counter laxatives, as some may not be safe during pregnancy. It is important to encourage them to consult with a healthcare provider before using any medications for this issue.

Proper positioning during pregnancy is another critical area of education, particularly in the later stages. Pregnant clients should avoid lying flat on their backs for extended periods, as this can compress the vena cava, a major vein responsible for returning blood to the heart. This compression can lead to reduced blood flow, causing discomfort, dizziness, or even more serious complications. Instead, clients should be encouraged to adopt side-lying positions, which improve circulation and reduce strain on the body.

Iron supplementation is frequently recommended during pregnancy to prevent anemia, a condition that can lead to fatigue and other complications if untreated. However, clients should be made aware of the potential side effects of iron supplementation, such as constipation, and provided with strategies to manage them. Encouraging the inclusion of high-iron foods, such as leafy greens, legumes, and lean meats, can complement supplementation and support healthy hemoglobin levels. Clients should also be advised to adhere to prescribed doses and report any persistent issues to their healthcare provider.

Recognizing Signs of Pregnancy

Educating clients about the signs of pregnancy is essential for ensuring they understand the progression of pregnancy and know when to seek medical attention. These signs are grouped into three categories: **presumptive**, **probable**, and **positive**, each providing varying levels of certainty about pregnancy.

Presumptive signs are the earliest indications and are subjective in nature. These include symptoms reported by the client, such as missed periods (amenorrhea), frequent urination, nausea, fatigue, and changes in skin pigmentation like darkening of the areolas or the appearance of linea nigra. While these signs suggest pregnancy, they are not definitive as they can also result from other conditions or hormonal changes.

Probable signs, on the other hand, are objective findings observed by a healthcare provider or detected through testing. These include a positive result on an over-the-counter pregnancy test, which indicates the presence of human chorionic gonadotropin (hCG) in the urine. Other probable signs include changes in the reproductive organs, such as the softening of the cervix (Goodell's sign), bluish discoloration of the vaginal mucosa (Chadwick's sign), and changes in uterine size and shape, which are typically identified during a physical examination.

Positive signs are the definitive indicators of pregnancy and confirm its presence beyond any doubt. These include detecting the fetal heartbeat using a Doppler device, visual confirmation of the fetus via ultrasound, and observing fetal movements during a clinical examination. Positive signs are critical for establishing the presence of a viable pregnancy and ruling out other potential conditions.

Clear communication about these signs helps clients understand what they can expect during pregnancy and when it is important to contact a healthcare provider. For example, clients should know that while presumptive and probable signs provide early clues, positive signs are necessary for confirmation. By fostering this understanding, healthcare providers empower clients to navigate the early stages of pregnancy with greater confidence and clarity, ensuring timely access to care when needed.

Supporting Clients with Multifetal Pregnancies

Supporting clients with multifetal pregnancies involves providing specialized care and education to address the increased complexity and risks associated with carrying more than one fetus. Multifetal pregnancies, including twins, triplets, and higher-order multiples, require heightened prenatal monitoring and tailored interventions to ensure the safety and well-being of both the mother and the fetuses.

Clients should be educated about the frequency of multifetal pregnancies. Twins occur in approximately **1 in 85 births**, while triplets are much rarer, occurring in about **1 in 8,100 births**. The likelihood of multifetal pregnancies increases with certain factors, including **advanced maternal age** (particularly in women over 35) and the use of **fertility treatments**, such as ovulation-inducing medications or assisted reproductive technologies like in-vitro fertilization (IVF). Understanding these factors helps clients contextualize their pregnancy and its unique demands.

A key concept in multifetal pregnancies is the distinction between **monozygotic (identical)** and **dizygotic (fraternal)** twins. Monozygotic twins result from a single fertilized egg that splits into two embryos, leading to identical genetic material. These twins may share a placenta (monochorionic) or, less commonly, amniotic sacs, which increases the risk of complications such as **twin-to-twin transfusion syndrome (TTTS)**. In contrast, dizygotic twins occur when two separate eggs are fertilized by two sperm, resulting in genetically distinct siblings. They typically have separate placentas (dichorionic) and amniotic sacs, which reduces some risks compared to monozygotic twins. Understanding these differences is crucial for guiding maternal and neonatal care plans.

Clients should be made aware of the increased risks associated with multifetal pregnancies. These include:

- **Preterm Labor and Birth**: The risk of preterm delivery rises significantly with the number of fetuses. Most twin pregnancies deliver around **36 weeks**, while triplets often deliver even earlier. Preterm birth can result in complications such as respiratory distress syndrome (RDS) or developmental delays in the neonates.
- **Gestational Diabetes**: The additional metabolic demands of carrying multiple fetuses increase the risk of developing gestational diabetes, which requires careful management to avoid complications.
- **Hypertensive Disorders**: Conditions like preeclampsia are more common in multifetal pregnancies and may require early delivery to protect maternal and fetal health.
- **Intrauterine Growth Restriction (IUGR)**: Restricted growth can occur when fetuses compete for nutrients and space, particularly in monochorionic pregnancies.

Early detection of multifetal pregnancies through **ultrasound** is vital for developing a comprehensive care plan. Regular ultrasounds are used to monitor fetal growth, amniotic fluid levels, and placental function. Clients should be educated on the importance of attending all scheduled prenatal visits, as these allow for early identification and management of potential complications. Additional tests, such as biophysical profiles or non-stress tests, may be required to assess fetal well-being, particularly in the third trimester.

A tailored care plan is essential for ensuring the health of both the mother and the fetuses. Nutritional counseling is critical, as mothers of multiples require increased caloric and protein intake to support fetal development. Encouraging adequate hydration, rest, and stress management is also important. For those at high risk of preterm labor, providers may recommend activity modifications, medications to reduce uterine contractions, or even hospitalization in severe cases.

In addition to medical care, emotional support and education are crucial for clients expecting multiples. The demands of a multifetal pregnancy can be overwhelming, and providing clear, compassionate guidance helps clients navigate the physical, emotional, and logistical challenges. Encourage clients to seek support from their healthcare team and connect with support groups or resources tailored to parents of multiples.

Educating Clients on Prenatal Physical Examinations

Educating clients about the importance of routine prenatal physical examinations is a vital part of promoting maternal and fetal health. These examinations provide critical insights into the progression of pregnancy and help identify any potential complications early, allowing for timely intervention. By understanding the purpose and scope of these assessments, clients can actively engage in their care and feel more confident during their visits.

Routine prenatal exams often begin with a **urinalysis**, a simple but essential test used to monitor glucose, protein, and ketones. Elevated glucose levels may indicate gestational diabetes, while the presence of protein can be an early sign of preeclampsia. Monitoring ketones can provide information about hydration and nutritional status. Explaining these tests to clients helps them appreciate their significance and reinforces the importance of regular prenatal visits.

Physical assessments are another key component of prenatal care. During each visit, providers may use **palpation and auscultation of the abdomen** to monitor fetal growth and well-being. Palpation allows the provider to estimate the size and position of the fetus, while auscultation with a Doppler device enables the detection of the fetal heartbeat, a moment that often reassures and excites clients. These non-invasive techniques provide valuable information about the pregnancy's progression and help detect potential issues, such as growth restrictions or abnormal fetal positions.

It is also important to address specific evaluations, such as **visual assessments of the cervix** or **rectal examinations**, which are typically deferred unless necessary. These more invasive assessments are usually reserved for cases where gynecologic concerns arise or during the later stages of pregnancy to evaluate labor readiness. Providing clear explanations about why and when such examinations might be performed can alleviate anxiety and help clients feel more comfortable with the process. Emphasizing that these evaluations are tailored to their individual needs fosters trust and ensures that clients view their care as personalized and respectful.

Educating clients about the components of prenatal examinations also involves explaining which assessments are typically included at various stages of pregnancy. For example, in the first trimester, the focus may be on confirming the pregnancy, dating it accurately through ultrasound, and establishing a baseline for the mother's health. In the second trimester, routine blood pressure monitoring and fetal growth assessments become more central, while the third trimester often involves closer monitoring for complications and preparation for delivery. This stage-specific approach helps clients understand the purpose behind each visit, reducing uncertainty and empowering them to participate actively in their care.

3.1.3 Postpartum Client Support

Providing effective postpartum support is a critical aspect of maternal care, ensuring a smooth transition for clients as they recover from childbirth. This care focuses on both the physical recovery of the mother and her emotional well-being, addressing the unique challenges of the postpartum period. For NCLEX-PN preparation, understanding the scope of postpartum care, common complications, and interventions is essential for delivering comprehensive and patient-centered nursing support.

Physical Recovery

After delivery, a client's body undergoes significant changes as it begins to heal and return to a pre-pregnancy state. Nurses play a key role in assisting with this recovery, including monitoring and managing symptoms, providing education on self-care, and identifying potential complications. Key aspects of physical recovery include:

- **Uterine Involution**: The uterus contracts to shrink back to its pre-pregnancy size. Clients may experience cramping, known as afterpains, especially during breastfeeding due to the release of oxytocin. Educating clients on what to expect and offering pain management strategies, such as warm compresses or prescribed medications, can provide relief.
- **Lochia**: Postpartum vaginal discharge, known as lochia, progresses through stages (rubra, serosa, and alba) as the uterus heals. Clients should be educated on the normal progression of lochia and when to seek medical attention for signs of abnormal bleeding, such as excessive clots or a foul odor.
- **Perineal Care**: For clients who experienced a vaginal delivery, particularly those with perineal tears or episiotomies, proper hygiene is essential to prevent infection. Educating clients on using a peri-bottle for cleaning, changing pads frequently, and recognizing signs of infection (e.g., swelling, redness, or discharge) helps ensure proper healing.

Pain management, whether related to a cesarean incision, perineal trauma, or general postpartum discomfort, is another critical component of care. Nurses should assess pain levels frequently, administer prescribed medications as needed, and educate clients on non-pharmacological methods, such as positioning and relaxation techniques, to manage discomfort effectively.

Emotional Well-Being

The emotional changes that occur postpartum are as significant as the physical ones. Hormonal shifts, fatigue, and the demands of caring for a newborn can lead to various emotional responses, ranging from the "baby blues" to postpartum depression.

- **Baby Blues**: Many clients experience mood swings, tearfulness, and irritability during the first few weeks postpartum. While these feelings are typically transient, nurses should offer reassurance and support, normalizing the experience while remaining vigilant for signs of more severe emotional distress.
- **Postpartum Depression (PPD)**: Unlike the baby blues, postpartum depression is more persistent and can significantly impact a client's ability to care for themselves or their baby. Educating clients on recognizing symptoms, such as prolonged sadness, feelings of hopelessness, or difficulty bonding with their newborn, is critical. Nurses should provide referrals to mental health resources and encourage open communication about emotional well-being.
- **Encouraging Support Systems**: Clients benefit from a strong support network, whether from family, friends, or community resources. Nurses can guide clients in seeking assistance with childcare, household responsibilities, and emotional support during the postpartum period.

Early Identification and Management of Complications

Promptly identifying complications is a cornerstone of postpartum care. Nurses should assess clients frequently for signs of common postpartum issues, including:

- **Postpartum Hemorrhage (PPH)**: Excessive bleeding, typically defined as more than 500 mL after a vaginal delivery or 1,000 mL after a cesarean, is a medical emergency. Signs include heavy bleeding, rapid heart rate, low blood pressure, and pallor. Immediate interventions may include uterine massage, administering medications such as oxytocin, and preparing for advanced medical procedures if necessary.
- **Infection**: Infections, such as endometritis, perineal wound infections, or mastitis, can develop postpartum. Educating clients to recognize signs like fever, chills, localized pain, or unusual discharge is vital. Nurses should provide guidance on preventive measures, such as proper hygiene and early breastfeeding support, while being prepared to administer antibiotics or other treatments as needed.
- **Thromboembolism**: The postpartum period carries an increased risk of deep vein thrombosis (DVT) and pulmonary embolism (PE). Clients should be educated on recognizing symptoms such as leg swelling, warmth, or sudden shortness of breath, and encouraged to engage in light physical activity to improve circulation.

Education on Self-Care

Teaching clients how to care for themselves during the postpartum period is a crucial aspect of support. Topics to include are:

- **Breast Care**: Whether breastfeeding or not, clients should be educated on managing engorgement, recognizing signs of mastitis, and using appropriate techniques to support lactation or suppress milk production.
- **Nutrition and Hydration**: A balanced diet rich in nutrients supports recovery and, for breastfeeding clients, enhances milk production. Adequate hydration is also critical, particularly for those nursing.
- **Physical Activity**: Clients should be encouraged to resume physical activity gradually, starting with light exercises such as walking, to promote circulation and overall well-being. Guidance on avoiding strenuous activities until cleared by a healthcare provider is also important.

Promoting Maternal-Infant Bonding

Encouraging early bonding between the client and the newborn is another essential aspect of postpartum care. Skin-to-skin contact, breastfeeding support, and teaching clients how to read and respond to their baby's cues foster a positive connection. Nurses should assess for any diffiiculties in bonding and provide resources or interventions to address challenges.

3.1.4 Comprehensive Care for Newborns (Birth–1 Month) and Infants/Toddlers

Providing comprehensive care for newborns and young infants involves addressing their immediate physical needs, fostering growth and development, and equipping parents with the knowledge and skills to care for their child confidently. This section outlines essential aspects of newborn and infant care, including feeding, hygiene, monitoring for health concerns, and promoting overall well-being.

Assisting with Feeding and Routine Neonatal Procedures

Feeding is a cornerstone of newborn care, whether the child is breastfed, formula-fed, or using a combination of both. Nurses must support parents in establishing safe and effective feeding practices. For breastfeeding parents, assistance with latching techniques, positioning, and understanding feeding cues is essential. Educating parents on the frequency of feedings—typically every 2–3 hours—and the importance of monitoring for adequate wet and soiled diapers ensures the newborn is receiving sufficient nutrition.

For formula-fed newborns, proper preparation and handling of formula are critical. Teach parents to carefully follow the manufacturer's instructions for mixing formula and to always use clean, sterilized bottles. Safe warming practices include using warm water or a bottle warmer, avoiding direct microwave heating to prevent hot spots, and always testing the temperature on the inner wrist before feeding. Parents should also be informed about safe storage practices, such as refrigerating prepared formula, discarding partially used bottles within 24 hours, and never mixing leftover formula with fresh batches. These steps reduce the risk of contamination and ensure the infant's safety.

Routine neonatal procedures, such as administering vitamin K injections and performing hearing screenings, are essential for the newborn's immediate health. Nurses should explain the purpose of these procedures to parents, ensuring they understand their importance in preventing complications like bleeding disorders and identifying early developmental issues.

Safe Practices for Umbilical Cord Care

Umbilical cord care is another crucial aspect of newborn care. Educate parents about keeping the cord clean and dry to prevent infection. Proper hand hygiene before and after handling the cord is vital. Parents should clean the area around the cord 3–4 times daily with a cotton swab and avoid using alcohol or antimicrobial solutions unless instructed by a healthcare provider. Diapers should be folded below the cord to allow air circulation and prevent moisture buildup, which can delay drying and separation.

Normal changes in the cord, such as darkening and eventual detachment, should be explained to parents, along with signs of potential infection. Advise them to contact a healthcare provider if they notice redness, swelling, foul odor, or discharge from the cord area. This guidance helps parents feel confident in managing this aspect of newborn care while knowing when to seek medical attention.

Managing Medical Conditions and Developmental Concerns

In some cases, newborns may have medical conditions or developmental concerns that require specialized care. For instance, infants with a cleft palate face unique challenges related to feeding and growth. Educate parents about the timing of surgical correction, typically performed between 8 and 12 months, and its importance for normal growth, language development, and facial appearance.

In the interim, parents should be taught about specialized feeding techniques and devices, such as bottles designed for infants with cleft palates, to ensure adequate nutrition. Nurses should monitor these infants for complications like speech delays or recurrent ear infections and coordinate with specialists for early interventions. Providing emotional support and connecting parents with resources, such as support groups, can also help them navigate these challenges with greater confidence.

Monitoring Growth, Development, and Parental Bonding

Ongoing monitoring of a newborn's growth and development is a key component of comprehensive care. Regular weight and length measurements, as well as head circumference assessments, help ensure the infant is growing appropriately. Parents should also be encouraged to track developmental milestones, such as visual tracking, cooing, and smiling, and to report any concerns to their healthcare provider.

Parental bonding is equally important during this period, as it lays the foundation for a secure attachment and healthy emotional development. Nurses can promote bonding by encouraging skin-to-skin contact, responsive feeding, and engaging parents in their infant's daily care routines.

Advocating for Immunizations and Preventive Measures

Preventive healthcare is critical in the newborn period. Educate parents on the importance of timely immunizations, beginning with the hepatitis B vaccine, which is typically administered shortly after birth. Highlight the role of vaccines in protecting their child from serious illnesses and discuss the recommended immunization schedule to help parents stay informed and proactive.

Additionally, preventive measures such as safe sleep practices reduce the risk of sudden infant death syndrome (SIDS). Teach parents to place their baby on their back to sleep, use a firm mattress without loose bedding, and avoid co-sleeping. Guidance on maintaining a smoke-free environment and regular handwashing further supports the infant's health and safety.

3.2 Pediatric and Adolescent Care

3.2.1 Meeting the Needs of Preschoolers and School-Age Children

Providing care for preschoolers and school-age children requires a developmental approach, recognizing their growing independence, social skills, and cognitive abilities. This stage of childhood, typically spanning ages 3 to 12, presents unique opportunities for fostering healthy growth, addressing developmental milestones, and educating families about essential health practices. Nurses must adapt their care strategies to the specific needs of this age group, ensuring effective communication, promoting safety, and supporting both physical and emotional development.

Developmentally Appropriate Care

At this stage, children are rapidly developing their language, reasoning, and motor skills. Nurses should adapt communication techniques to match the child's age and understanding. For preschoolers, this may involve using simple, concrete language and incorporating play therapy to reduce fear and build trust. Play becomes a powerful tool for assessment and teaching, allowing nurses to observe developmental milestones while engaging the child in a comforting and familiar activity.

For school-age children, who are more capable of understanding abstract concepts, providing clear explanations about procedures and involving them in their care fosters a sense of control and reduces anxiety. Encouraging questions and addressing their concerns openly helps build confidence and trust.

Promoting Injury Prevention

Injury prevention is a key focus during this stage, as children become more active and explore their environment. Educating parents and caregivers about common safety risks is essential.

Topics to address include:

- **Home Safety:** Emphasize the importance of childproofing, including securing furniture, covering electrical outlets, and storing hazardous materials out of reach.
- **Outdoor Safety:** Encourage helmet use during activities such as biking, skating, or riding scooters and discuss the importance of supervising children during play.
- **Water Safety:** Highlight the need for constant supervision around pools or other bodies of water, and stress the importance of swimming lessons for older children.
- **Car Safety:** Educate families about appropriate car seats or booster seats based on the child's age, height, and weight, and reinforce the importance of seat belt use.

Nutrition and Immunizations

Proper nutrition is critical for growth and development during these years. Nurses should educate families on providing balanced meals that include a variety of fruits, vegetables, whole grains, lean proteins, and dairy products. Address common concerns such as picky eating in preschoolers or the increased appetite and nutritional needs of school-age children as they approach adolescence. Encouraging healthy snacking and limiting sugary or processed foods supports both overall health and dental hygiene.

Immunizations remain a cornerstone of preventive care. Review the recommended immunization schedule for this age group, which includes vaccines such as DTaP, MMR, varicella, and influenza. Emphasize the importance of staying up-to-date with vaccinations to protect against serious diseases and promote community health.

Assessing and Monitoring Developmental Milestones

Regular assessment of developmental milestones is crucial for identifying potential delays or concerns. In addition to physical growth, evaluate motor skills, language development, social interactions, and cognitive abilities. For preschoolers, milestones include activities like hopping, drawing simple shapes, and forming complete sentences. For school-age children, milestones shift toward academic achievements, problem-solving skills, and forming peer relationships.

Physical development also includes monitoring for changes in body proportions and dental health. Educate parents about the typical timeline for primary tooth eruption, which generally begins around **6 months of age**. By age 3, most children will have a full set of 20 primary teeth. Use simple methods to help families understand expected dental progress, such as subtracting **6** from the child's age in months to estimate the number of teeth for children under 2 years old (e.g., an 18-month-old child is expected to have around **12 teeth**).

Discuss normal variations in dental development, such as delayed eruption or spacing issues, and educate parents on the importance of regular dental visits starting around the first birthday or within six months of the first tooth eruption. Emphasize the role of fluoride in preventing cavities and provide guidance on proper brushing techniques for young children. For school-age children, highlight the transition from primary teeth to permanent dentition, which typically begins around age 6, and discuss the importance of orthodontic evaluations if needed.

Recognizing When to Refer

Variations in physical, developmental, or dental milestones are often normal but may occasionally indicate underlying concerns. Nurses should educate families on recognizing when further evaluation is necessary, such as if a child:

- Has not achieved expected motor or language milestones for their age.
- Displays persistent difficulties in social interactions or behavior.
- Shows significant delays in dental development, such as no teeth by age 1.
- Experiences chronic dental issues, including frequent cavities or abnormal tooth placement.

By identifying these concerns early and facilitating appropriate referrals, nurses help ensure timely interventions and improved outcomes for children.

3.2.2 Providing Care for Adolescents

Adolescence is a critical period of growth and development marked by significant physical, emotional, and social changes. Nurses providing care to adolescents must address the unique challenges and needs of this age group, ensuring a holistic approach that supports both physical health and mental well-being. Adolescents are navigating the transition from childhood to adulthood, which includes developing a sense of identity, managing peer relationships, and coping with the pressures of school, family, and social life.

Addressing Psychosocial and Physical Changes

During adolescence, the body undergoes rapid growth and hormonal changes that impact physical and emotional health. Nurses should approach adolescents with sensitivity, fostering open communication and building trust to encourage honest discussions about their concerns. Adolescents may face challenges such as body image issues, peer pressure, and struggles with self-esteem. Providing reassurance and normalizing these experiences can help them navigate this transitional period.

Mental health is another critical area of focus. Adolescents are at an increased risk of developing anxiety, depression, and other mental health conditions. Nurses should promote healthy coping mechanisms, such as exercise, journaling, and seeking support from trusted adults. Educating adolescents on recognizing signs of mental health concerns, like persistent sadness, irritability, or withdrawal from activities, empowers them to seek help when needed. Referrals to mental health professionals or school counselors may be necessary for more severe cases.

Education on Common Physical Conditions

Adolescents, especially those involved in sports and physical activities, are prone to certain growth-related conditions, such as **Osgood-Schlatter disease**. This condition is characterized by inflammation of the patellar tendon at its attachment to the tibia and is commonly seen in physically active adolescents during periods of rapid growth.

Cause and Symptoms

Osgood-Schlatter disease occurs due to repetitive stress on the knee, typically from activities like running, jumping, or squatting. The condition is most common in adolescents aged 10 to 15 years and is more likely to occur during growth spurts when bones, muscles, and tendons are rapidly developing. Symptoms include:

- Knee pain, often worse during or after physical activity.
- Swelling or tenderness below the kneecap.
- A visible or palpable bony bump at the site of inflammation.

Prevention and Management

Preventing Osgood-Schlatter disease involves encouraging proper warm-up routines, stretching, and avoiding overtraining or repetitive strain on the knees. Adolescents should be educated on the importance of listening to their bodies and taking breaks when experiencing discomfort.

For those experiencing symptoms, management strategies include:

- Rest and avoiding activities that exacerbate pain.
- Applying ice to reduce swelling and alleviate discomfort.
- Over-the-counter pain relievers, such as ibuprofen or acetaminophen, if recommended by a healthcare provider.
- Physical therapy to strengthen the surrounding muscles and improve flexibility.

Adolescents and their caregivers should be advised to seek medical attention if symptoms persist or worsen, as untreated cases can lead to chronic discomfort and functional limitations.

Promoting Injury Prevention

Injury prevention is essential for adolescents, particularly those engaged in sports or other physical activities. Nurses should educate adolescents on the importance of using proper protective gear, such as helmets, knee pads, and appropriate footwear, to reduce the risk of injury. Emphasizing the role of warm-ups, cool-downs, and stretching in preventing sprains, strains, and other musculoskeletal issues is also critical.

For adolescent athletes, ensuring a balanced training regimen with adequate rest days can help prevent overuse injuries. Encouraging cross-training and varying activities can reduce repetitive strain on specific muscle groups while promoting overall fitness.

Supporting Proper Nutrition

Nutrition plays a vital role in supporting the rapid growth and increased physical activity of adolescents. Nurses should educate adolescents on the importance of consuming a balanced diet rich in fruits, vegetables, whole grains, lean proteins, and dairy products. Adolescents often face nutritional challenges, such as skipping meals, consuming excessive processed or sugary foods, and experimenting with restrictive diets due to body image concerns.

Highlighting the benefits of proper nutrition for energy, muscle development, and overall health can motivate adolescents to make healthier choices. Special attention should be given to ensuring adequate calcium and vitamin D intake to support bone health during peak growth periods.

Immunizations and Preventive Health

Adolescence is a critical time for ensuring immunizations are up-to-date. Nurses should review the recommended immunization schedule, which includes vaccines like:

- **Tetanus, diphtheria, and acellular pertussis (Tdap)**.
- **Meningococcal vaccines** to protect against meningitis.
- **Human papillomavirus (HPV) vaccine** to reduce the risk of HPV-related cancers.
- **Annual influenza vaccine** to protect against seasonal flu.

In addition to vaccines, adolescents should be encouraged to engage in regular preventive health practices, such as annual check-ups, vision and dental screenings, and discussions about reproductive health. Nurses should provide age-appropriate education on topics like safe sex practices, sexually transmitted infections (STIs), and contraception, ensuring the information is delivered in a nonjudgmental and supportive manner.

Fostering Independence and Responsibility

As adolescents strive for independence, nurses should encourage them to take an active role in their health. Teaching them how to manage their medications, schedule appointments, and recognize when to seek medical attention fosters autonomy and prepares them for the transition to adulthood. Open, respectful communication and a focus on empowering the adolescent to make informed decisions about their health are critical components of care.

3.2.3 Comparing Clients to Developmental Milestones

Monitoring a child's development is a fundamental aspect of pediatric care, ensuring that they are meeting expected milestones and identifying any delays or concerns early. Developmental milestones provide benchmarks for evaluating progress in areas such as motor skills, cognitive abilities, and social interactions. When milestones are not met, timely recognition and intervention can significantly improve outcomes for the child. For nurses, understanding normal growth patterns, recognizing signs of delays, and educating caregivers are essential components of providing comprehensive care.

Recognizing Normal Growth Patterns

Growth and development follow predictable sequences, but the timing of milestones can vary slightly among children. Nurses should be familiar with critical motor milestones, such as pulling to a standing position by **11–12 months** and walking independently by **15 months**. Cognitive and social milestones, such as imitating actions, forming simple words, and interacting with caregivers, should also be assessed regularly.

While variations in the timing of these milestones may not always indicate a problem, consistent delays warrant further evaluation. For example, a child who is unable to sit without support by 9 months or who has not begun walking by 18 months may require additional assessment to determine the underlying cause.

Educating Caregivers About Developmental Delays

Caregivers play a key role in monitoring their child's development. Educating them about the signs of potential delays empowers them to seek help early. Key indicators to discuss include:

- **Gross Motor Delays**: Difficulty sitting, crawling, standing, or walking within the expected timeframes.
- **Fine Motor Delays**: Challenges with tasks like grasping objects or transferring items between hands.
- **Language Delays**: Limited babbling by 9 months, lack of single words by 16 months, or difficulty forming two-word phrases by 24 months.
- **Social or Emotional Delays**: Limited eye contact, inability to respond to their name, or lack of interest in interacting with caregivers or peers.

When caregivers express concerns, nurses should validate their observations and provide guidance on next steps, including referrals for developmental screenings or specialist evaluations.

Promoting Developmental Monitoring

Routine developmental screenings are essential in pediatric care, serving as a proactive measure to monitor a child's progress and identify potential concerns early. These screenings assess various domains of development, including motor skills, language, cognitive abilities, and social-emotional behaviors. Tools like the **Ages and Stages Questionnaire (ASQ)** and the **Denver Developmental Screening Test** are widely used and help healthcare providers pinpoint specific areas where a child may need additional support or further evaluation. These tools involve input from caregivers, making them a collaborative approach to understanding a child's developmental trajectory.

Educating caregivers about the value of regular **well-child visits** and the developmental assessments conducted during these visits is critical. These checkups not only allow for physical health monitoring, such as growth measurements and immunizations, but also provide opportunities to address developmental milestones. Caregivers who understand the importance of these visits are more likely to adhere to the recommended schedule and actively participate in their child's care.

In addition to formal screenings, engaging caregivers in activities that promote development is a vital part of preventive care. For infants, encouraging **tummy time** helps strengthen the neck, shoulders, and core muscles, preparing them for milestones like rolling over, sitting, and crawling. For toddlers and older children, **interactive play** activities, such as reading books, playing with building blocks, and singing songs, support cognitive and language development while fostering parent-child bonding.

Nurses play a key role in empowering caregivers by offering practical guidance tailored to their child's developmental stage. For instance, advising caregivers to create a stimulating environment with age-appropriate toys, encourage problem-solving through play, and model language by narrating daily activities helps promote healthy development. Nurses should also address potential barriers, such as time constraints or lack of resources, by suggesting simple, low-cost activities that fit into the family's routine.

Furthermore, when caregivers express concerns about their child's development, nurses should provide reassurance and validate their observations while emphasizing the importance of follow-up evaluations when necessary. This collaborative approach builds trust and ensures caregivers feel supported in their role, ultimately enhancing the child's developmental outcomes. By combining formal screenings with practical, everyday strategies, healthcare providers can create a comprehensive framework for nurturing a child's growth and ensuring they reach their full potential.

3.3 Adult and Older Adult Care

3.3.1 Clients Ages 18–64 Years

Providing care for clients between the ages of 18 and 64 encompasses addressing the diverse health needs and challenges faced by adults in this broad age group. This life stage is often characterized by varied lifestyles, occupational demands, and stressors, requiring a flexible and individualized approach to care. Nurses play a vital role in promoting health, preventing illness, and supporting clients in managing the physical and emotional transitions that occur during this phase of life.

Promoting Self-Care and Preventive Measures

Encouraging self-care and adherence to preventive health measures is essential for maintaining well-being in adulthood. Nurses should educate clients on the importance of regular health screenings, including:

- **Cancer Screenings**: Annual or biennial mammograms starting at age 40–50, routine Pap smears for cervical cancer prevention, and colonoscopies beginning at age 45 (or earlier based on risk factors).
- **Chronic Disease Monitoring**: Routine blood pressure checks, cholesterol screenings, and diabetes testing to identify and manage risk factors early.

- **Lifestyle Interventions**: Counseling on proper nutrition, regular exercise, adequate sleep, and stress management techniques to support overall health.

Educating clients about immunizations is another critical aspect of preventive care. Adults should remain up-to-date on vaccines, including the annual influenza vaccine, tetanus booster every 10 years, and specific vaccines such as the shingles vaccine for those over 50 and the pneumococcal vaccine for individuals with certain risk factors. Nurses should emphasize that preventive measures not only improve individual health outcomes but also reduce the burden of chronic illnesses on families and communities.

Addressing Hormonal Transitions: Perimenopause and Menopause

Hormonal changes during perimenopause and menopause significantly impact many clients in this age group, particularly those assigned female at birth. Perimenopause typically begins in the mid-40s, with menopause officially marked by the absence of menstruation for 12 consecutive months, often occurring around age 50–52. These transitions involve complex physiological and emotional changes, requiring comprehensive care and support.

Physiological Changes

Clients may experience a wide range of symptoms, including irregular menstrual cycles, hot flashes, night sweats, vaginal dryness, and changes in libido. These symptoms result from fluctuating and declining estrogen levels. Nurses should educate clients about these changes, normalizing the experience and addressing misconceptions about menopause.

Emotional Well-Being

In addition to physical symptoms, clients may face mood swings, anxiety, and depression during this transition. These emotional changes can be compounded by life stressors, such as career demands, caregiving responsibilities, and personal health concerns. Nurses should assess for signs of emotional distress, provide reassurance, and, when necessary, refer clients to mental health professionals or support groups.

Hormone Replacement Therapy (HRT): Benefits and Risks

Hormone replacement therapy (HRT) is a common treatment option for managing moderate to severe menopausal symptoms. Nurses should educate clients on the potential benefits of HRT, such as relief from hot flashes, improved sleep quality, and prevention of osteoporosis. However, it is equally important to discuss the risks associated with HRT, including an increased risk of blood clots, stroke, breast cancer, and cardiovascular events.

When considering HRT, nurses must assess for contraindications, such as:

- A history of **unexplained vaginal bleeding.**
- A personal or family history of **stroke**, **breast cancer**, or **blood clots.**
- Active or recent history of **liver disease.**

Clients should be guided to weigh the benefits and risks of HRT in consultation with their healthcare provider. Nurses should also educate clients about non-hormonal alternatives for managing symptoms, such as medications, lifestyle modifications, and natural remedies, to ensure a well-rounded approach to care.

Lifestyle Adjustments for Long-Term Health

Supporting clients through menopause involves more than symptom management; it also requires addressing long-term health risks associated with hormonal changes. Nurses should encourage lifestyle adjustments that promote bone health, cardiovascular health, and overall well-being. These include:

- **Calcium and Vitamin D Intake:** Educating clients on consuming adequate amounts of calcium and vitamin D through diet or supplements to reduce the risk of osteoporosis.
- **Regular Weight-Bearing Exercise:** Activities like walking, jogging, and strength training help maintain bone density and muscle strength.
- **Heart-Healthy Practices:** Encouraging a diet rich in fruits, vegetables, whole grains, and healthy fats, along with routine exercise, helps mitigate the increased cardiovascular risks associated with menopause.

Managing Symptoms to Enhance Quality of Life

Clients often struggle with symptoms such as **hot flashes**, **night sweats**, and **sleep disturbances** that significantly impact their quality of life. Nurses should provide practical strategies for managing these symptoms, such as:

- Dressing in lightweight, layered clothing to manage temperature fluctuations.
- Keeping a cool environment at night and using breathable bedding materials.
- Practicing relaxation techniques, such as yoga or meditation, to reduce stress and improve sleep.
- Staying hydrated and avoiding known triggers for hot flashes, such as caffeine, spicy foods, and alcohol.

For vaginal dryness, nurses can recommend over-the-counter lubricants or vaginal moisturizers and discuss the potential use of localized estrogen treatments for severe cases, ensuring clients are aware of their options.

Providing Holistic Support

Nurses should take a holistic approach to care, recognizing that each client's experience of menopause and midlife varies. Providing emotional support, creating space for open conversations, and offering individualized care plans empower clients to navigate this life stage with confidence. Encouraging regular follow-ups and fostering trust strengthens the nurse-client relationship and ensures that care is responsive to changing needs.

3.3.2 Clients Ages 65 and Over

Providing care for clients aged 65 and over requires a nuanced approach that addresses the physical, emotional, and social challenges associated with aging. This population often experiences a combination of chronic illnesses, functional limitations, and age-related changes that require comprehensive care strategies. Nurses play a pivotal role in promoting independence, improving quality of life, and ensuring that care is patient-centered and responsive to the unique needs of older adults.

Addressing the Complexities of Aging

Aging is a natural process that brings about significant physiological changes in every system of the body, often increasing the risk of developing chronic illnesses. Conditions such as hypertension, diabetes, osteoarthritis, and heart disease are particularly common in older adults and frequently occur simultaneously. This combination of coexisting illnesses complicates care, requiring a nuanced and individualized approach to management. For nurses preparing for the NCLEX-PN, it is essential to understand the unique challenges these conditions present and the interventions needed to support older clients effectively.

Managing chronic illnesses in older adults requires a combination of education, monitoring, and collaboration. Nurses must guide clients in understanding their conditions and taking an active role in their care. For example, clients with diabetes need education on blood glucose monitoring, meal planning, and foot care to prevent complications such as neuropathy or infections. Similarly, managing hypertension involves promoting adherence to medications, educating clients on the importance of a low-sodium diet, and encouraging regular physical activity. Clients with osteoarthritis may require strategies to manage joint pain and improve mobility, such as engaging in low-impact exercises, maintaining a healthy weight, and using assistive devices like braces or walkers to reduce strain on joints. These strategies not only improve physical health but also enhance clients' confidence and independence.

Polypharmacy is another critical issue in the care of older adults. Many clients take multiple medications, which increases the risk of drug interactions, side effects, and non-adherence. Nurses play a pivotal role in reviewing medication regimens regularly, monitoring for adverse effects, and educating clients about proper medication use. Collaboration with healthcare providers is essential to simplify regimens when possible, reducing the burden on clients while maintaining the effectiveness of treatments. Educating clients about potential interactions between prescription medications, over-the-counter drugs, and supplements is equally important in minimizing risks.

Functional limitations are another common challenge among older adults, as physical decline can impact mobility, vision, hearing, and the ability to perform daily activities. These limitations often reduce quality of life and increase the risk of falls and injuries. Nurses should assess clients for fall risks, identify specific limitations, and recommend interventions such as the use of assistive devices like canes or walkers. Occupational therapy can be particularly beneficial for clients struggling with daily activities, as it helps them regain independence and improve safety in their living environments. Preventing falls is a priority, and nurses can provide practical advice, such as ensuring adequate lighting, removing tripping hazards, and installing grab bars in bathrooms.

Promoting Independence and Quality of Life

While aging may bring challenges, nurses can help clients maintain independence and a high quality of life by addressing their physical, emotional, and social needs. **Geriatric assessments** are an essential tool for identifying areas where support is needed, evaluating physical health, cognitive function, emotional well-being, and social resources.

- **Activities of Daily Living (ADLs):** Assessing a client's ability to perform tasks such as bathing, dressing, eating, and mobility provides insight into their functional status. When limitations are identified, nurses can recommend resources like home health aides or adaptive equipment to support independence.
- **Instrumental Activities of Daily Living (IADLs):** Tasks such as managing finances, preparing meals, and using transportation are critical for independent living. Nurses should evaluate these abilities and connect clients with community resources or family support if assistance is needed.

Promoting independence also involves fall prevention, a major concern for older adults. Nurses should educate clients and caregivers on strategies to reduce fall risks, such as:

- Ensuring homes are free of hazards like loose rugs or poor lighting.
- Encouraging the use of non-slip footwear and grab bars in bathrooms.
- Promoting regular exercise to improve balance, strength, and coordination.

Supporting Emotional and Social Well-Being

The emotional and social aspects of aging are equally as important as physical health, yet they are often overlooked in healthcare settings. Older adults frequently encounter challenges that can significantly impact their quality of life, such as social isolation, depression, and anxiety. These issues may arise due to a variety of factors, including the loss of loved ones, retirement, reduced mobility, or limited access to social opportunities. Recognizing and addressing these challenges is a vital part of holistic care, as emotional well-being is closely linked to overall health.

Nurses play a crucial role in assessing older clients for signs of emotional distress. This involves not only observing behavioral changes, such as withdrawal, irritability, or a lack of interest in activities, but also engaging clients in open, empathetic conversations to understand their experiences and concerns. When emotional distress is identified, providing targeted support can make a significant difference in enhancing a client's quality of life.

Encouraging participation in social activities or senior programs can be particularly effective in combating social isolation. These programs provide opportunities for older adults to engage with peers, build relationships, and participate in meaningful activities that foster a sense of belonging and purpose. Whether it's joining a local walking group, attending community center events, or engaging in hobbies, these connections can alleviate feelings of loneliness and improve emotional health.

Recommending mental health resources is another critical aspect of support. Therapy, whether individual or group-based, can provide older clients with the tools to manage depression or anxiety. Support groups tailored to specific experiences, such as grief or chronic illness, offer a space for clients to share their feelings and learn from others facing similar challenges. Nurses should normalize seeking mental health support and work to reduce any stigma clients may feel about accessing these resources.

Grief and loss are common experiences for older adults, whether due to the death of a spouse, friends, or even the loss of physical abilities and independence. Navigating these changes can be overwhelming, and nurses must approach this aspect of care with compassion and sensitivity. Offering a listening ear, providing referrals to grief counselors or support groups, and helping clients find ways to honor their loved ones or adapt to new circumstances are all valuable interventions.

Preventive Health and Wellness

Preventive care remains important in older adults to maintain health and detect issues early. Nurses should educate clients about recommended screenings and preventive measures, including:

- **Cancer Screenings:** Mammograms, colorectal cancer screenings, and prostate exams may still be relevant depending on the client's overall health and life expectancy.
- **Bone Health:** Bone density testing for osteoporosis is critical, particularly for postmenopausal clients or those with a history of fractures.
- **Vaccinations:** Older adults should receive vaccines such as the influenza vaccine annually, the pneumococcal vaccine, and the shingles vaccine to reduce the risk of severe infections.

Lifestyle modifications also play a significant role in promoting wellness. Nurses should encourage older adults to:

- Stay physically active through low-impact activities like walking, yoga, or swimming.
- Maintain a balanced diet rich in nutrients to support energy, bone health, and immune function.
- Prioritize adequate sleep and stress reduction techniques to enhance overall well-being.

Palliative and End-of-Life Care

For older adults with advanced illnesses or declining health, palliative and end-of-life care become essential components of nursing practice. Nurses should focus on providing comfort, managing symptoms, and supporting clients and their families through this process. Key aspects include:

- **Pain and Symptom Management:** Ensuring clients are free from pain and discomfort, using both pharmacological and non-pharmacological interventions.
- **Advance Care Planning:** Encouraging discussions about advance directives, living wills, and healthcare proxies to honor the client's wishes.
- **Emotional and Spiritual Support:** Offering compassionate care to address the emotional and spiritual needs of clients and their families during this time.

3.3.3 Assisting Clients with Expected Life Transitions

Life transitions are inevitable as clients progress through various stages of adulthood, and these changes often have profound physical, emotional, and social impacts. Nurses play a vital role in supporting clients as they navigate these transitions, offering guidance, resources, and empathy to help them adapt to new circumstances. Whether the transition involves a career change, retirement, or assuming the role of a caregiver, or it is prompted by health-related challenges such as starting dialysis or entering long-term care, clients benefit greatly from personalized care that addresses their unique needs and concerns.

One of the most common transitions clients face is retirement, which, while often anticipated with excitement, can also bring challenges. For many, retirement signifies a loss of routine, social connections, or a sense of purpose, which can contribute to feelings of isolation or depression. Nurses can help clients prepare for this major life change by encouraging them to explore new hobbies, volunteer opportunities, or part-time work to stay engaged and maintain a sense of fulfillment. Additionally, nurses should assess clients for emotional challenges during this time and provide referrals to mental health resources or social programs if needed.

For some clients, transitions may involve taking on the role of a caregiver for an aging parent, a spouse, or even a grandchild. This responsibility can be rewarding but also emotionally and physically demanding, leading to caregiver stress or burnout. Nurses should provide education on setting boundaries, accessing community support services, and seeking respite care to alleviate the burden of caregiving. Encouraging caregivers to prioritize their own well-being through regular self-care practices is essential for maintaining their health and effectiveness in the role.

Health-related transitions, such as the need for dialysis, are particularly challenging and often require significant adjustments to a client's lifestyle and daily routine. Starting dialysis can be overwhelming, as it involves frequent treatments, dietary changes, and emotional adaptation to the reality of chronic illness. Nurses should focus on education, helping clients understand the dialysis process, manage dietary restrictions, and recognize the importance of adhering to their treatment schedule. Emotional support is equally critical, as clients may feel a loss of independence or struggle with the long-term implications of their condition. Open communication and a supportive approach can ease these feelings and empower clients to take an active role in their care.

Similarly, transitioning to long-term care is a significant life event that often involves a mixture of emotions for clients and their families. Clients may experience feelings of loss, fear, or uncertainty about moving into a facility, while families may grapple with guilt or concern over the decision. Nurses in these settings should approach this transition with sensitivity, focusing on building trust and fostering a sense of belonging. Providing clients with a clear understanding of what to expect in long-term care and involving them in decisions about their daily routines can help them regain a sense of control. Family members should also be supported with education about the facility's services and regular updates on their loved one's well-being.

Throughout all these transitions, effective coping strategies are essential for maintaining emotional and physical health. Nurses can guide clients in developing skills such as stress management, problem-solving, and setting realistic goals. Encouraging clients to access social support networks, whether through family, friends, or community groups, is another important strategy for fostering resilience. When necessary, referrals to mental health professionals, social workers, or spiritual care providers can offer additional layers of support.

3.4 Collecting and Interpreting Health Data

Collecting and interpreting health data is a cornerstone of effective nursing care, enabling nurses to assess a client's condition, identify potential concerns, and develop individualized care plans. This process involves gathering comprehensive health histories, conducting thorough physical assessments, and utilizing evidence-based practices to ensure accurate and meaningful interpretation of findings. By combining clinical expertise with a systematic approach to data collection, nurses can make informed decisions that improve client outcomes and enhance overall care delivery. For NCLEX-PN preparation, mastering these skills is essential to providing competent, patient-centered nursing care across diverse settings.

3.4.1 Gathering Health Histories and Baseline Physical Data

Gathering comprehensive health histories and establishing baseline physical data are fundamental components of nursing care. These steps provide the foundation for creating individualized care plans and ensuring effective client management. Nurses must employ skilled interviewing techniques, conduct thorough physical examinations, and integrate evidence-based practices (EBP) into clinical care to achieve the best outcomes for their clients.

The process begins with a client interview, which requires active listening, empathy, and the use of open-ended questions to encourage clients to share detailed and accurate information. Nurses should create a comfortable environment that fosters trust, as this promotes more open communication. By using questions tailored to the client's situation, such as inquiries about their medical history, lifestyle, and current concerns, nurses can uncover vital information that informs the assessment process. For example, asking about a client's family history of chronic illnesses, current medications, and any recent changes in health status provides critical context for understanding their overall condition.

Following the interview, nurses conduct an initial physical examination to gather objective data. This includes measuring vital signs, such as blood pressure, heart rate, respiratory rate, and temperature, as well as performing a head-to-toe assessment. During this process, nurses observe for any abnormalities, palpate areas of concern, and document findings accurately. Thorough documentation is essential for creating a clear record of the client's baseline status, which serves as a reference point for future evaluations and interventions. Consistent and accurate documentation also ensures effective communication among the healthcare team, reducing the risk of errors or omissions.

Incorporating evidence-based practice into patient assessments and interventions enhances the quality of care provided. Evidence-based practice (EBP) is the integration of the best available research evidence with clinical expertise and patient preferences. Unlike best practices or standard-based approaches, which may rely solely on tradition or institutional policies, EBP emphasizes the use of current research to guide clinical decisions. For example, evidence-based guidelines might inform the management of a client with hypertension by recommending specific diagnostic tests, lifestyle interventions, and medication protocols tailored to their individual needs.

Educating healthcare providers about EBP is an important step in improving patient outcomes. Nurses should advocate for the integration of research findings into everyday practice, highlighting how evidence-based interventions have been shown to reduce complications, improve recovery times, and enhance client satisfaction. At the same time, it is crucial to consider individual client circumstances and preferences when applying these guidelines. For instance, a client's cultural beliefs or financial constraints may influence their willingness or ability to adhere to certain recommendations, and these factors must be respected and addressed in the care plan.

Teaching strategies must also be adapted to align with the abilities and preferences of each client. This requires nurses to assess a client's level of health literacy, preferred learning style, and readiness to learn. For example, visual aids or hands-on demonstrations may be more effective for some clients than written materials. Ensuring that education is delivered in a manner the client can understand and apply empowers them to take an active role in managing their health.

3.4.2 Identifying Barriers to Communication and Learning

Effective communication and education are essential components of nursing care, yet various barriers can impact a client's ability to understand and comply with instructions. Nurses must be adept at recognizing and addressing these barriers, which may include language differences, cultural considerations, sensory impairments, cognitive limitations, or a lack of prior knowledge about health topics. By tailoring teaching strategies to meet individual needs, nurses can foster better understanding, encourage compliance, and ultimately improve client outcomes.

One of the most common barriers to communication is **language differences**, which can lead to misunderstandings and reduced compliance with care plans. Clients who are not fluent in the primary language of their healthcare provider may struggle to follow instructions or express their concerns. Nurses should prioritize the use of professional interpreters when needed and provide written materials in the client's preferred language to enhance comprehension. It is equally important to avoid using family members as interpreters, as this may compromise accuracy and privacy.

Cultural factors can also influence communication and learning. Clients may have cultural beliefs or practices that affect their perceptions of health and illness, preferred treatment methods, or willingness to ask questions. Nurses must approach these differences with sensitivity and respect, using culturally competent care strategies to build trust and foster collaboration. For example, understanding a client's cultural views on medication adherence or dietary restrictions can help nurses design education plans that align with their values while still meeting clinical goals.

Clients with **sensory or cognitive impairments** may face additional challenges in processing information. A client with hearing loss, for instance, may benefit from written instructions or visual aids, while a client with visual impairments might require audio recordings or large-print materials. For clients with cognitive limitations, such as those with dementia or developmental delays, nurses should use simple, concrete language, repeat key points as needed, and verify understanding through teach-back methods. Adapting the pace and delivery of education to the client's abilities ensures that they can retain and apply the information effectively.

To optimize learning, nurses should sequence instruction from the **least complex to the most complex**. For example, when teaching a client about managing diabetes, begin with foundational concepts such as recognizing symptoms of hypo- and hyperglycemia before moving on to more advanced topics like insulin injection techniques. This gradual progression helps clients build confidence and understanding as they master each step.

Using **clear, plain language** is another critical strategy. Avoiding overly technical or medically oriented terms makes the information accessible and reduces confusion. For example, instead of saying "hypertension," use the term "high blood pressure" and explain its effects in simple terms. This approach ensures that clients can connect the information to their own experiences and apply it in their daily lives.

It is also important to **assume limited prior knowledge** about the topic, particularly for complex medical conditions or procedures. Building on foundational concepts allows clients to form a strong base of understanding. For instance, when educating a client about the importance of medication adherence, start by explaining the condition being treated and how the medication works, then proceed to specifics about dosage and timing.

Active participation enhances comprehension and retention. Nurses should address the client directly, ensuring they are the primary focus of the conversation, while involving family members or caregivers only when appropriate and in line with the client's preferences. This empowers the client to take ownership of their care and fosters a sense of autonomy. Providing **examples, visuals, or demonstrations** further reinforces understanding. For instance, demonstrating how to use an inhaler or showing a video on proper wound care can make abstract instructions more tangible and easier to remember.

Finally, creating an environment where clients feel comfortable asking questions is crucial for reinforcing understanding. Encouraging open dialogue and clarifying doubts not only ensures compliance but also strengthens the nurse-client relationship. Nurses should actively invite questions and confirm understanding through techniques such as teach-back, where the client repeats the instructions in their own words. This approach helps identify gaps in knowledge and provides an opportunity for further clarification.

3.5 Promoting Community Connections and Preventive Care

Promoting community connections and preventive care is essential for fostering health and well-being across diverse populations. Nurses play a pivotal role in linking clients to local resources, encouraging healthy behaviors, and emphasizing the importance of preventive measures to reduce the risk of illness and complications. By addressing social determinants of health, advocating for community involvement, and guiding clients toward proactive health management, nurses contribute to building stronger, healthier communities. This section highlights strategies for integrating community-based resources and preventive care into nursing practice, equipping clients with the tools they need to maintain optimal health.

3.5.1 Identifying Community Resources for Clients

One of the most impactful ways nurses can support clients is by connecting them with community resources that enhance their ability to achieve and maintain health goals. Whether addressing medical, emotional, or social needs, leveraging community services ensures clients have access to comprehensive care beyond the clinical setting. Nurses play a vital role in bridging the gap between healthcare and community support by identifying resources tailored to each client's unique circumstances, evaluating their accessibility, and empowering clients to utilize them effectively.

Connecting clients with local services begins with understanding their specific needs and challenges. For clients managing chronic illnesses, referrals to **home health agencies** can provide access to skilled nursing care, physical therapy, or medication management within the comfort of their homes. These services not only improve health outcomes but also reduce the risk of hospitalization. Similarly, for clients facing emotional or mental health concerns, **counseling services** or support groups offer a safe space to navigate issues such as anxiety, depression, or grief. Nurses should also consider social determinants of health, such as housing instability or food insecurity, and connect clients to programs like housing assistance or local food banks.

Evaluating the affordability and accessibility of programs is crucial in ensuring their effectiveness. Nurses should consider financial barriers clients may face, such as a lack of insurance coverage or limited income, and prioritize referrals to programs offering low-cost or free services. For example, federally funded clinics, sliding-scale counseling services, and nonprofit organizations can provide essential care at reduced costs. Accessibility also includes factors like location, transportation, and availability of services. If a client lacks reliable transportation, nurses might explore options like telehealth services, mobile clinics, or community organizations offering rides to appointments.

Another important consideration is cultural and language appropriateness. Community resources should align with the client's cultural background, values, and language preferences to ensure comfort and effectiveness. For instance, a client whose primary language is not English may benefit from being referred to bilingual service providers or programs that offer translation services. This not only enhances understanding but also fosters trust and engagement.

Nurses can also empower clients by providing detailed information about the resources available to them. This includes explaining what services are offered, how to access them, and what to expect when engaging with these programs. For instance, a nurse helping a client enroll in a smoking cessation program might provide an overview of the program's structure, such as whether it includes group sessions, one-on-one counseling, or pharmacological support, and help the client understand how it aligns with their goals.

Beyond connecting clients to existing services, nurses serve as advocates for improving community health resources. By identifying gaps in care, such as a lack of mental health services in a rural area or long wait times for affordable housing programs, nurses can work collaboratively with local organizations and policymakers to address these deficiencies. Advocacy efforts ensure that communities continue to evolve and provide robust support for their residents.

3.5.2 Recognizing Clients in Need of Immunizations

Immunizations are one of the most effective tools in preventive healthcare, protecting individuals and communities from potentially life-threatening diseases. As a nurse, recognizing clients in need of immunizations requires a proactive approach to screening, education, and follow-up care. Ensuring clients are up-to-date on their vaccinations not only safeguards their health but also contributes to broader public health efforts by reducing the spread of infectious diseases. For NCLEX-PN preparation, understanding the principles of vaccination screening, education, and follow-up is critical for providing safe and evidence-based care.

Screening for vaccination status is the first step in identifying clients in need of immunizations. Nurses should review the client's health history, focusing on their age, medical conditions, lifestyle, occupation, travel history, and potential exposure to infectious diseases. For example, children and adolescents should follow the CDC-recommended immunization schedule, which includes vaccines such as DTaP, MMR, varicella, and HPV. Adults may need vaccines like the annual influenza vaccine, Tdap, or shingles vaccine, depending on their age and risk factors. Older adults, particularly those over 65, should be assessed for pneumococcal vaccines and other age-appropriate immunizations.

Risk factors play a critical role in determining the need for additional or earlier vaccinations. Clients with chronic illnesses such as diabetes, heart disease, or lung conditions may require certain vaccines sooner than the general population due to their increased susceptibility to complications. Similarly, immunocompromised clients, such as those undergoing chemotherapy or living with HIV, may need modified vaccination schedules. Pregnant clients should also be assessed for vaccines like Tdap to protect both the mother and the newborn from pertussis. Nurses must remain vigilant for these factors and ensure their recommendations are tailored to the individual client's health status.

Providing education about disease prevention is a vital part of the immunization process. Clients may have concerns or misconceptions about vaccines, such as fears of side effects or misinformation about their safety. Nurses should address these concerns with evidence-based information, explaining how vaccines work, their role in preventing disease, and the minimal risks associated with them compared to the benefits. For instance, educating a client about the importance of the annual flu vaccine might include discussing how influenza can lead to severe complications, especially in older adults or those with chronic conditions, and how the vaccine significantly reduces this risk.

When educating clients, it is essential to use clear and accessible language, avoiding overly technical terms. Nurses should also provide specific guidance on what to expect after vaccination, such as common side effects like mild soreness at the injection site or low-grade fever, and when to seek medical attention for rare but serious reactions. Encouraging clients to ask questions and addressing their doubts fosters trust and promotes compliance with vaccination recommendations.

Follow-up care is another important component of immunization management. Many vaccines require multiple doses for full protection, such as the HPV vaccine or the hepatitis B series. Nurses should emphasize the importance of completing the entire series and provide reminders or scheduling assistance to ensure clients return for subsequent doses. For clients receiving vaccines with recommended boosters, such as the tetanus vaccine, maintaining accurate records and offering timely reminders helps keep them protected.

In addition to individual client care, nurses contribute to public health by advocating for herd immunity through vaccination. This collective immunity protects vulnerable populations, such as infants, the elderly, and those who cannot receive vaccines due to medical conditions. Nurses should encourage clients to view immunizations not only as a personal health measure but also as a way to safeguard their families and communities.

3.5.3 Participating in Health Screenings and Promotion Programs

Health screenings and promotion programs are essential components of preventive care, enabling the early detection of chronic conditions and fostering a culture of wellness within communities. Nurses play a pivotal role in organizing and participating in these activities, using their expertise to guide individuals toward healthier lifestyles while emphasizing the value of holistic health. For NCLEX-PN preparation, understanding the nurse's responsibilities in health screenings and promotion is crucial for delivering comprehensive, proactive care.

Health screenings are an effective way to identify potential health issues before they develop into serious conditions. Nurses often assist in organizing or conducting activities such as **blood pressure checks**, **blood glucose tests**, **vision screenings**, and **cholesterol monitoring** at community events, workplaces, or wellness fairs. These programs provide convenient access to preventive care, particularly for individuals who may not regularly visit a healthcare provider. Nurses must ensure that screenings are conducted accurately and efficiently, interpreting results when appropriate and referring clients for further evaluation as needed. For instance, identifying elevated blood pressure during a screening could prompt a referral to a primary care provider for hypertension management, potentially preventing complications like heart disease or stroke.

Advocating for regular health screenings is another key responsibility for nurses. Early detection of chronic conditions such as **diabetes, hypertension, and hyperlipidemia** allows for timely interventions that can improve outcomes and reduce healthcare costs. Nurses should educate clients about the importance of routine check-ups and screenings based on age, risk factors, and family history. For example, recommending annual mammograms for women over 40 or colonoscopies starting at age 45 aligns with evidence-based guidelines and underscores the importance of proactive health management.

Health promotion programs extend beyond screenings to focus on empowering individuals and communities to achieve optimal well-being. Nurses can educate clients on the **World Health Organization's (WHO)** definition of health, which emphasizes a state of complete physical, mental, and social well-being—not merely the absence of disease or infirmity. This holistic perspective encourages clients to view health as a dynamic, multidimensional concept that encompasses physical fitness, emotional resilience, and social connectedness.

In health promotion activities, nurses should clarify that these initiatives support overall well-being but are not the definition of health itself. For example, participating in an exercise class or attending a mental health workshop are activities that contribute to achieving well-being but do not solely define what it means to be healthy. This distinction helps clients understand the broader scope of health while emphasizing the value of adopting proactive measures to maintain it.

Encouraging a **proactive approach to health maintenance** is at the core of health promotion. Nurses should guide clients and communities in integrating wellness practices that address all aspects of health. This might include:

- **Physical Health**: Promoting regular physical activity, balanced nutrition, and adequate sleep as fundamental components of a healthy lifestyle.
- **Mental Health**: Encouraging mindfulness practices, stress management techniques, and access to mental health resources to build emotional resilience.
- **Social Health**: Supporting community engagement, social connections, and healthy relationships to enhance a sense of belonging and purpose.

Nurses can also collaborate with community leaders, schools, and workplaces to implement health promotion initiatives tailored to specific populations. For instance, offering smoking cessation workshops, weight management programs, or stress reduction seminars targets common health concerns and encourages participants to take ownership of their well-being.

Participating in health screenings and promotion programs also provides an opportunity for nurses to advocate for underserved populations. Addressing barriers such as limited access to healthcare, lack of transportation, or language differences ensures that these programs are inclusive and accessible to all. Nurses can work to identify gaps in care and collaborate with local organizations to expand resources and services to those in need.

3.5.4 Encouraging High-Risk Behavior Prevention

Preventing high-risk behaviors is a critical component of nursing care, particularly in the context of promoting long-term health and reducing the prevalence of preventable diseases. High-risk behaviors such as smoking, excessive alcohol consumption, and substance abuse significantly increase the likelihood of developing chronic conditions, including cardiovascular disease, liver dysfunction, and certain cancers. Nurses play an essential role in educating clients about these risks, supporting behavior change, and guiding them toward healthier lifestyle choices.

One of the most impactful areas of high-risk behavior prevention is **smoking cessation**. Tobacco use is a leading cause of preventable deaths and is linked to a range of serious health conditions, including lung cancer, chronic obstructive pulmonary disease (COPD), and heart disease. Nurses should provide evidence-based counseling on the benefits of quitting smoking, emphasizing the immediate and long-term health improvements, such as better lung function, reduced risk of heart attack, and improved quality of life. Supportive interventions might include connecting clients to smoking cessation programs, recommending nicotine replacement therapies, and helping clients set achievable goals to quit.

Alcohol moderation is another important focus area. Excessive alcohol consumption can lead to liver damage, high blood pressure, and mental health issues. Educating clients on what constitutes moderate drinking—defined by the CDC as up to one drink per day for women and up to two drinks per day for men—helps them make informed decisions about alcohol use. For clients struggling with alcohol dependence, nurses should offer nonjudgmental support, provide referrals to counseling or rehabilitation programs, and collaborate with healthcare teams to develop a comprehensive treatment plan.

Substance abuse prevention and education are crucial, particularly for at-risk populations such as adolescents, individuals with a family history of addiction, or those in high-stress environments. Nurses should educate clients on the dangers of substance use, including its impact on physical and mental health, and offer resources for treatment when needed. Open, empathetic communication is key to building trust and encouraging clients to seek help without fear of stigma or judgment.

Promoting healthy lifestyle choices is equally important in preventing high-risk behaviors and fostering overall well-being. Nurses should provide **nutritional guidance** tailored to each client's needs, including education on daily caloric intake based on age, gender, and activity level. For example, **sedentary older men**, **active adult women**, and **children** generally require around **2000 calories per day**, while more active individuals may need additional calories to support their energy expenditure. A balanced **2000-calorie diet** typically includes:

- **6 ounces of grains** (preferably whole grains), such as bread, rice, or pasta.
- **2½ cups of vegetables**, including a variety of colors and types like leafy greens, carrots, and broccoli.
- **2 cups of fruits**, emphasizing fresh or minimally processed options like apples, berries, or oranges.
- **3 cups of dairy**, such as milk, yogurt, or cheese, or equivalent calcium-fortified alternatives.

Providing specific examples of meals or snacks that align with these guidelines helps clients visualize and implement healthy eating habits. For instance, a balanced breakfast might include whole-grain toast with avocado, a boiled egg, and a side of mixed berries, while a healthy dinner could feature grilled chicken, roasted vegetables, and quinoa.

Nurses should also emphasize the importance of **regular screenings and assessments** to detect nutritional deficiencies or imbalances. Identifying issues like low iron levels, vitamin D deficiencies, or elevated cholesterol early allows for targeted interventions that can prevent chronic conditions such as anemia, osteoporosis, or heart disease. Screening tools such as food diaries, blood tests, and body composition analysis can provide valuable insights into a client's nutritional status and guide personalized care plans.

Encouraging a proactive approach to health maintenance involves educating clients about the broader benefits of a healthy lifestyle, including increased energy, improved mental clarity, and enhanced emotional well-being. Nurses should foster a supportive environment where clients feel empowered to ask questions, seek guidance, and make gradual, sustainable changes to their habits. Recognizing that behavior change is a process, nurses can celebrate small victories with clients, reinforcing their progress and motivating them to continue.

3.5.5 Nonpharmacological Techniques and Preventive Interventions

Nonpharmacological techniques and preventive interventions are increasingly recognized as effective tools for managing a variety of health conditions and enhancing overall well-being. These approaches offer clients alternative or complementary options to traditional treatments, empowering them to take an active role in their health management. Nurses play a critical role in introducing and educating clients about these techniques, ensuring they understand their applications, benefits, and potential integration into existing care plans.

One prominent nonpharmacological method is **biofeedback**, a scientifically backed technique that uses electronic monitoring devices to help clients gain control over certain physiological functions. Through biofeedback, clients learn to consciously influence bodily processes such as heart rate, blood pressure, muscle tension, and even body temperature. By observing real-time data on a monitor, clients can identify and adjust their responses to stressors, achieving a greater sense of control over their physical and emotional well-being. For example, biofeedback has been effectively used to help clients manage **stress**, **chronic pain**, and **anxiety** by teaching them to reduce muscle tension or lower their heart rate through relaxation techniques.

Applications of biofeedback extend to various conditions. Clients with migraines can use biofeedback to identify and mitigate triggers by relaxing specific muscle groups, reducing the frequency and intensity of their headaches. Similarly, individuals with hypertension may benefit from biofeedback by learning to lower their blood pressure through controlled breathing and mindfulness. Even clients with chronic conditions such as fibromyalgia or irritable bowel syndrome (IBS) can find relief by using biofeedback to regulate symptoms influenced by stress.

Biofeedback is particularly valuable as a **complement to traditional treatments**, offering clients a noninvasive and drug-free option to enhance their care plans. While it does not replace the need for medications or other medical interventions, it serves as a powerful adjunct for improving quality of life and promoting autonomy. Nurses should educate clients on the availability of biofeedback programs, which may be offered through community health centers, wellness clinics, or private practitioners. By guiding clients toward these resources, nurses help them access evidence-based interventions that align with their preferences and goals.

When discussing biofeedback, it is useful to compare it with other **nonpharmacological methods**, such as meditation, visualization, and mindfulness-based stress reduction (MBSR). While biofeedback focuses on measurable physiological regulation using electronic monitoring, techniques like meditation and visualization rely on cultivating a sense of mental calm and focus. For instance, meditation encourages clients to quiet the mind and reduce stress through deep breathing and mindfulness, while visualization involves imagining calming or positive scenarios to achieve relaxation. Both methods are effective for reducing stress and promoting mental health, but they lack the real-time feedback provided by biofeedback, which allows clients to see and adjust their physiological responses in a concrete way.

Nurses should emphasize that biofeedback and other nonpharmacological techniques are **highly individualized** and can be tailored to suit a client's specific needs and conditions. For clients who prefer a more structured and data-driven approach, biofeedback might be an ideal choice. On the other hand, clients seeking low-cost or self-guided practices may benefit from meditation or visualization, which can be practiced independently with minimal resources. Encouraging clients to experiment with multiple methods helps them discover what works best for their unique situation.

In addition to biofeedback and mindfulness techniques, other nonpharmacological interventions include yoga, tai chi, acupuncture, and progressive muscle relaxation. Each of these methods offers distinct benefits, ranging from improving flexibility and strength to reducing stress and promoting overall well-being. Nurses should be familiar with these options to provide well-rounded education and support to clients exploring complementary therapies.

3.6 Ensuring Safety and Compliance

Ensuring safety and compliance is a fundamental responsibility for nurses, encompassing the implementation of measures to protect clients from harm and promote adherence to care plans. This involves identifying potential risks, educating clients on safe practices, and fostering an environment that supports understanding and cooperation. By addressing safety concerns and encouraging compliance with treatments and interventions, nurses play a vital role in improving health outcomes and enhancing the overall quality of care. This section focuses on strategies to uphold safety standards and ensure client compliance in diverse healthcare settings, a critical competency for NCLEX-PN success.

3.6.1 Monitor for Potential Hazards

Monitoring for potential hazards is an essential component of nursing care, ensuring that clients are protected from preventable harm in all aspects of their lives. Nurses must remain vigilant in identifying and addressing risks associated with environmental safety, medication adherence, and lifestyle factors. These efforts not only safeguard clients' health but also contribute to building a foundation for long-term well-being and compliance with care plans. For NCLEX-PN preparation, mastering the principles of hazard identification and mitigation equips nurses to provide safe, effective, and client-centered care.

One critical area of focus is **environmental safety**, which involves assessing the client's surroundings to minimize risks of injury or harm. This is particularly important for vulnerable populations, such as older adults or individuals with mobility challenges, who may be at greater risk of falls or accidents. Nurses should evaluate the client's home environment for hazards such as loose rugs, inadequate lighting, or cluttered walkways that could lead to trips and falls. Recommending modifications, like installing grab bars in bathrooms, using non-slip mats, and ensuring clear pathways, helps create a safer living space. For clients in healthcare settings, ensuring that call bells are within reach, bedrails are appropriately used, and medical equipment is functioning correctly are essential practices for maintaining safety.

Medication adherence is another critical area where hazards can arise. Clients may face challenges in managing their medications, including forgetting doses, misunderstanding instructions, or experiencing side effects that deter compliance. Nurses must assess for these risks by conducting thorough medication reconciliations, reviewing the client's prescriptions, and identifying potential drug interactions or duplications. Educating clients on the purpose, dosage, and timing of each medication, as well as addressing common side effects, fosters better understanding and adherence. For clients with complex regimens, recommending tools such as pill organizers or setting reminders on mobile devices can simplify the process and reduce the risk of errors.

In addition to understanding medications, clients need to be aware of potential risks related to **over-the-counter drugs** or supplements, which may interact with their prescribed treatments. Nurses should encourage open communication about all substances the client is taking, emphasizing the importance of consulting healthcare providers before adding new products to their regimen. This proactive approach prevents unintended consequences and promotes safer medication practices.

Lifestyle factors also play a significant role in client safety. Behaviors such as smoking, excessive alcohol consumption, poor dietary habits, or a lack of physical activity can increase the risk of chronic conditions and exacerbate existing health issues. For example, a client with hypertension who consumes a high-sodium diet may experience complications such as stroke or heart failure. Nurses should provide tailored education on the importance of adopting healthier habits, offering practical recommendations like reducing salt intake, increasing physical activity, and managing stress through relaxation techniques. For clients who engage in high-risk behaviors, such as substance abuse, nurses should address these concerns with empathy and provide referrals to appropriate support programs or counseling services.

Monitoring for hazards also extends to assessing the client's mental and emotional well-being. Stress, anxiety, or depression can impact safety by contributing to forgetfulness, poor decision-making, or neglect of self-care. Nurses should remain attentive to signs of emotional distress and provide resources, such as mental health counseling or support groups, to help clients manage these challenges.

In all aspects of monitoring, effective communication is key. Nurses should encourage clients to voice their concerns and ask questions about their care. Building a trusting relationship fosters openness, making it easier to identify potential hazards and address them collaboratively. Additionally, involving family members or caregivers in safety discussions ensures that everyone in the client's support network is informed and equipped to assist.

3.6.2 Managing Postoperative and Post-Procedure Care

Postoperative and post-procedure care is a critical phase in a client's recovery, requiring attentive nursing interventions and comprehensive education to ensure optimal healing and prevent complications. Nurses play a pivotal role in guiding clients and their caregivers through this phase, addressing both physical and emotional needs, and promoting adherence to rehabilitation protocols. Effective postoperative care involves a combination of pain management, progressive rehabilitation exercises, education on potential complications, and emotional support.

A key component of postoperative care is providing **detailed guidance on recovery protocols** specific to the surgical procedure performed. For instance, clients recovering from a **mastectomy** require targeted interventions to restore mobility, promote circulation, and prevent complications such as lymphedema. Nurses should educate clients on the importance of beginning with **progressive rehabilitation exercises** tailored to their recovery stage. The initial exercise, such as squeezing a soft ball with the hand on the affected side, serves to promote circulation, prevent lymphedema, and build strength gradually in the arm. This simple yet effective activity lays the groundwork for more advanced exercises as the client regains strength.

As recovery progresses, nurses should guide clients on transitioning to more advanced exercises, such as **walking the hand up a wall**, gently **combing their hair**, or performing light stretches to improve range of motion. These activities help restore functional mobility, reduce stiffness, and encourage confidence in using the affected arm. Nurses must emphasize the importance of pacing these exercises according to the client's tolerance, ensuring that movements are pain-free and gradual to avoid strain or injury.

Pain management is another critical aspect of postoperative care. Clients often experience varying degrees of discomfort after surgery, and nurses should work collaboratively with the healthcare team to implement an effective pain management plan. This may include prescribed analgesics, non-pharmacological methods such as relaxation techniques or cold therapy, and education on proper medication use to prevent overuse or underuse. Teaching clients to communicate openly about their pain levels allows for timely adjustments to their care plan.

Addressing **scar care and emotional well-being** is also essential, particularly for clients coping with procedures like mastectomy that involve visible physical changes. Nurses should provide education on proper wound care to minimize infection risk and support optimal healing. Gentle scar massage, as advised by a healthcare provider, can improve tissue flexibility and reduce adhesions. Equally important is offering emotional support to clients as they adjust to changes in their body image and self-esteem. Referrals to counseling, support groups, or peer networks can provide valuable resources for clients navigating these psychological challenges.

Educating clients and caregivers on recognizing **signs of complications** is a vital preventive measure. Nurses should clearly outline symptoms that warrant immediate attention, such as signs of infection (e.g., redness, warmth, or discharge at the surgical site), excessive swelling, or impaired mobility in the affected limb. Providing guidance on when to contact a healthcare provider ensures that complications are addressed promptly, reducing the risk of further issues.

Multidisciplinary teams are instrumental in supporting a client's recovery and promoting adherence to rehabilitation protocols. Nurses should highlight the roles of physical therapists, occupational therapists, social workers, and dietitians in creating a holistic recovery plan. For example, physical therapists may design an individualized exercise program to enhance mobility and strength, while social workers can assist with navigating financial or logistical challenges related to follow-up care.

To ensure compliance with prescribed protocols, nurses must foster a collaborative relationship with clients and caregivers. This involves explaining the rationale behind each aspect of the care plan, addressing any concerns or misconceptions, and encouraging active participation in the recovery process. For example, demonstrating exercises during a follow-up visit or using visual aids to explain scar care techniques can boost the client's confidence and understanding.

Postoperative and post-procedure care is a multifaceted process that requires a balance of technical expertise, clear communication, and compassionate support. By focusing on progressive rehabilitation, pain management, complication prevention, and emotional well-being, nurses can empower clients to achieve a successful recovery. For NCLEX-PN preparation, mastering these principles ensures nurses are equipped to provide safe, evidence-based, and client-centered care during this critical phase of healing.

Chapter 4
Psychosocial Integrity

In the healthcare setting, psychosocial integrity plays a crucial role in providing holistic, client-centered care. This chapter focuses on the essential skills and knowledge needed to address the emotional, social, and psychological needs of clients. From fostering effective communication to managing emotional crises, understanding cultural values, and promoting self-esteem, psychosocial integrity encompasses a wide range of practices that ensure clients feel heard, respected, and supported throughout their healthcare journey.

As you prepare for the NCLEX-PN exam, this chapter will guide you through key concepts such as therapeutic communication, client and caregiver education, managing barriers to care, and culturally inclusive practices. By mastering these topics, you'll not only enhance your ability to meet client needs but also increase your confidence in handling complex psychosocial situations in your nursing career.

4.1 Educating Caregivers and Families on Behavioral Disorders

Caregivers and families serve as the foundation of emotional and psychological support for individuals with behavioral disorders. Their role becomes even more crucial when managing the needs of infants and children, especially those diagnosed with chronic conditions such as Hemophilia. Nurses, therefore, play a vital role in equipping caregivers with the knowledge and skills necessary to create environments that foster healthy psychosocial development. This chapter delves into the importance of educating caregivers about the psychosocial aspects of chronic conditions and providing practical strategies to help them manage their caregiving roles effectively.

4.1.1 The Impact of Altered Family Processes on Development

When families encounter stress, whether due to a chronic illness diagnosis or shifts in caregiving responsibilities, the repercussions can ripple through the entire family unit. Infants, for example, are particularly sensitive to disruptions in their environment because their psychosocial development heavily relies on the establishment of trust during the earliest stages of life. Erik Erikson's theory of psychosocial development identifies "trust versus mistrust" as the foundational stage for healthy emotional growth. Inconsistent caregiving, emotional withdrawal, or heightened stress levels within the family can disrupt the development of trust, leaving lasting effects on a child's relational patterns.

For instance, a family dealing with a Hemophilia diagnosis may experience fear, uncertainty, or guilt, which can influence how caregivers interact with the child. A caregiver's heightened anxiety may lead to overprotectiveness or inconsistent responses to the child's needs, potentially undermining the infant's ability to develop secure attachments. Therefore, educating caregivers about the importance of consistency and responsiveness is crucial in mitigating these effects and fostering a stable foundation for the child's emotional development.

4.1.2 The Role of Caregivers in Supporting Psychosocial Development

Caregivers play an indispensable role in a child's psychosocial development, acting as the primary architects of their emotional environment. Their behavior, responses, and interactions with the child shape not only the child's immediate emotional state but also their long-term psychosocial outcomes. A child's sense of security, trust, and ability to navigate the world begins within the caregiving relationship. This makes the creation of a supportive and nurturing environment critical, particularly for children managing behavioral disorders or chronic conditions.

A supportive environment is not solely about fulfilling a child's physical needs, such as feeding, bathing, and ensuring medical care; it also involves fostering emotional well-being. Caregivers must recognize how their own emotional states, actions, and responses directly influence the child's mental health and overall development. For instance, consistent, empathetic care builds a foundation of trust, while inconsistent or emotionally distant caregiving can hinder the child's ability to form secure attachments and develop resilience. This is particularly significant in children with conditions like Hemophilia, where the stress of managing the condition can add an additional layer of complexity to caregiving.

Understanding the Emotional Impact of Chronic Conditions

Chronic conditions like Hemophilia bring unique challenges to caregiving. While medical management is crucial, the psychosocial dimensions of these conditions often require equal attention. Children with chronic illnesses may face limitations that influence their daily lives, self-perception, and social interactions. For caregivers, these realities can lead to feelings of fear, guilt, or inadequacy, which can inadvertently affect how they respond to the child's needs.

For example, caregivers might become overprotective, limiting the child's ability to explore and develop independence. Conversely, some caregivers may emotionally withdraw due to stress or fear of doing something wrong, which can leave the child feeling isolated or misunderstood. Nurses play a vital role in helping caregivers understand these dynamics and guiding them to maintain a balanced approach that supports the child's physical and emotional needs without overcompensation or neglect.

Creating Predictable and Emotionally Safe Environments

One of the most powerful tools caregivers can provide is a predictable and emotionally safe environment. Predictability offers children a sense of stability, which is particularly valuable for those dealing with the uncertainties of chronic conditions. A structured environment with consistent routines helps children feel secure and reduces the anxiety that can arise from unpredictability.

Caregivers must also strive to model calm and composed behavior, especially during moments of stress or medical emergencies. Children are highly attuned to the emotions of their caregivers and often mirror their responses. For example, if a caregiver remains calm during a medical procedure, the child is more likely to feel reassured and cooperative. Nurses can teach caregivers techniques to manage their own stress, such as deep breathing or mindfulness exercises, which in turn benefits the emotional atmosphere they create for the child.

Empathy and Emotional Stability in Caregiving

Empathy is a cornerstone of effective caregiving. When caregivers respond empathetically to a child's emotions—whether it's fear, frustration, or sadness—they validate the child's experiences and foster a sense of security. This is especially important for children with chronic conditions, who may experience emotions that they cannot fully articulate. A caregiver who listens without judgment and provides reassurance helps the child feel understood and supported.

Furthermore, caregivers must be encouraged to maintain their own emotional stability. Chronic caregiving responsibilities can be overwhelming, and caregivers often neglect their own needs in the process. Nurses can educate caregivers on the importance of self-care, offering strategies such as setting boundaries, seeking respite care, or engaging in activities that bring them joy and relaxation. Caregivers who take care of themselves are better equipped to provide consistent and loving care to their children.

The Nurse's Role in Caregiver Support

Nurses are uniquely positioned to act as both educators and advocates for caregivers. By offering resources, emotional support, and practical strategies, nurses empower caregivers to feel confident in their roles. For instance, providing clear explanations about the child's condition, treatment plan, and expected outcomes helps caregivers feel more in control and less overwhelmed. Additionally, nurses can connect caregivers with community support networks, such as parent groups or counseling services, where they can share experiences and gain reassurance.

Ultimately, a caregiver's ability to create a stable, nurturing environment is not only a reflection of their own resilience but also a critical determinant of the child's psychosocial health. Through education, encouragement, and partnership, nurses can help caregivers navigate the complexities of their roles while ensuring that both the child's and the family's holistic needs are met.

4.1.3 Educating Caregivers About Chronic Conditions

Empowering caregivers begins with providing them with comprehensive education that addresses both the medical and emotional aspects of chronic conditions. Chronic illnesses not only affect the individual diagnosed but also ripple through family dynamics, introducing added responsibilities, financial stress, and emotional strain. Education tailored to the unique challenges of each family is essential for helping caregivers navigate these complexities while maintaining a nurturing and supportive environment for the child.

When caregivers understand the full scope of a chronic condition, they are better equipped to manage the demands of caregiving with confidence and empathy. Nurses play a vital role in this process by breaking down medical jargon, addressing fears, and equipping caregivers with the knowledge they need to make informed decisions. Education is not just about imparting facts—it is about helping families feel more in control, fostering resilience, and building a foundation of trust between the healthcare team and the family.

For example, explaining the nature of a chronic condition is a crucial first step. Providing caregivers with clear and detailed information about the progression, treatment options, and expected outcomes of a condition demystifies the diagnosis and alleviates fear of the unknown. Whether it is clarifying treatment timelines or discussing the potential challenges ahead, this knowledge empowers caregivers to plan for the future and respond proactively rather than reactively. Nurses must also address caregivers' questions and concerns openly, fostering an atmosphere of collaboration and understanding.

Equally important is helping caregivers recognize the behavioral and emotional impacts of chronic conditions on children. Chronic illnesses can influence a child's mood, behavior, and development, often leading to frustration, withdrawal, or fear. Without guidance, caregivers may misinterpret these changes, potentially responding in ways that exacerbate the child's distress. Educating caregivers on these behavioral impacts helps them adopt constructive approaches to address their child's emotional needs. For instance, if a child becomes irritable due to physical discomfort or limitations, caregivers can be guided to respond with patience and empathy, rather than frustration. This not only eases the child's distress but also reinforces a strong emotional bond between the caregiver and the child.

Another critical aspect of caregiver education is exploring the influence of family dynamics. Chronic conditions place considerable emotional and logistical strain on families, and the stress experienced by caregivers can inadvertently affect the child's emotional health. For example, a caregiver who is overwhelmed or anxious may unknowingly project those emotions onto the child, creating an atmosphere of tension or fear. Nurses can help caregivers identify these patterns and adopt healthier coping mechanisms, such as setting boundaries, seeking support, or using stress management techniques. By doing so, caregivers can create a more stable and supportive environment that promotes the child's overall well-being.

Providing caregivers with education is only part of the equation; it is equally important to create a safe space for them to express their concerns and receive emotional support. Caregiving can often feel isolating, and the emotional toll it takes can lead to burnout or feelings of inadequacy. Nurses can facilitate connections between caregivers and resources that provide emotional and practical support. This might include counseling services to address specific challenges, peer support groups where caregivers can share experiences and advice, or community programs that offer respite care or financial assistance. These resources not only alleviate some of the burden on caregivers but also remind them that they are not alone in their journey.

4.1.4 Practical Strategies for Caregivers

Caregivers often need actionable strategies to help them navigate the complexities of their roles effectively. Nurses can provide the following practical guidance:

1. **Creating a Stable Environment:**
   Encourage caregivers to establish consistent routines, as predictability helps children feel secure. A stable environment can mitigate the anxiety and emotional turbulence that often accompany chronic conditions.

2. **Promoting Positive Interactions:**
   Train caregivers to reinforce positive behaviors through praise, encouragement, and affection. Positive interactions not only strengthen the caregiver-child bond but also boost the child's self-esteem.

3. **Responding to Emotional Needs:**
   Teach caregivers to identify and respond appropriately to their child's emotional cues, such as frustration, sadness, or discomfort. Empathy and active listening are vital in building trust and emotional resilience.

4. **Managing Caregiver Stress:**
   Highlight the importance of self-care for caregivers. Suggest stress management techniques like mindfulness, physical activity, or seeking respite care when needed. Stressed caregivers are less able to provide the consistent, loving care that children require.

5. **Accessing Support Networks:**
   Encourage caregivers to build a network of family, friends, or professional support to share caregiving responsibilities and reduce feelings of isolation.

4.2 Therapeutic Approaches for Psychosocial Support

Psychosocial support is a cornerstone of holistic nursing care, addressing the emotional, psychological, and social needs of clients. By employing therapeutic approaches such as reminiscence therapy, validation therapy, reality orientation, and group sessions, nurses can improve client engagement, foster emotional well-being, and enhance the overall quality of care. These methods are not just tools but opportunities to build meaningful connections with clients, addressing their unique challenges in a compassionate and structured manner. The integration of foundational nursing theories further enriches these interventions, providing a robust framework for delivering effective psychosocial care.

Reminiscence Therapy

Reminiscence therapy encourages clients, particularly older adults, to reflect on and share memories from their past. This approach is especially effective for individuals with dementia or depression, as it helps them reconnect with meaningful experiences and regain a sense of identity. By discussing life events, achievements, or cherished moments, clients often experience improved mood, reduced feelings of isolation, and enhanced cognitive function. Nurses play a vital role in facilitating these sessions by creating a safe and supportive environment where clients feel comfortable sharing personal stories. For example, using photographs or music from the client's youth can stimulate recall and encourage interaction.

Validation Therapy

Validation therapy focuses on empathizing with clients' feelings and experiences, particularly when they are experiencing confusion or disorientation. This approach is commonly used with individuals who have dementia, as it emphasizes validating their emotions rather than challenging their perception of reality. For instance, if a client believes they are waiting for a long-deceased family member, the nurse might engage with the client's emotions rather than correcting the factual inaccuracy. This reduces agitation, builds trust, and fosters a sense of dignity for the client.

Reality Orientation

Reality orientation involves gently reorienting clients to the present time, place, and situation. This technique is particularly beneficial for individuals with cognitive impairments, such as those recovering from brain injuries or experiencing early stages of dementia. By using cues like calendars, clocks, and verbal reminders, nurses can help clients regain a sense of stability and reduce confusion. For example, a nurse might say, "Good morning, Mr. Johnson. Today is Monday, and it's time for your breakfast." This not only supports cognitive function but also reinforces a sense of routine and security.

Group Sessions

Group therapy provides clients with a structured environment to share their experiences, challenges, and successes with others facing similar issues. These sessions can address a variety of psychosocial needs, from managing anxiety to building social skills. For instance, group sessions for individuals coping with grief may focus on sharing personal stories, exploring coping mechanisms, and developing a supportive network. Nurses can facilitate these sessions by fostering open communication, ensuring inclusivity, and guiding the group toward productive outcomes. Research consistently demonstrates that group therapy enhances emotional resilience, reduces feelings of isolation, and promotes a sense of belonging.

4.2.1 Foundational Nursing Theories in Psychosocial Support

The practice of psychosocial support is deeply rooted in foundational nursing theories, which provide evidence-based frameworks for understanding and addressing clients' needs. These theories emphasize the importance of the nurse-client relationship, goal setting, problem-solving, and holistic care.

Hildegard Peplau's Interpersonal Relations Model

Peplau's theory underscores the therapeutic potential of the nurse-client relationship. She identified four phases—orientation, identification, exploitation, and resolution—that guide the nurse and client through a collaborative process of healing. For instance, during the orientation phase, the nurse builds trust by actively listening and empathizing with the client's concerns. This model is particularly relevant in therapeutic approaches such as validation therapy, where establishing rapport is essential for success.

Faye Glenn Abdellah's Twenty-One Nursing Problems

Abdellah's framework emphasizes identifying and addressing specific nursing problems, many of which are psychosocial in nature. For example, addressing a client's fear or anxiety is central to therapeutic interventions like reminiscence therapy or group sessions. By categorizing client needs into distinct areas, Abdellah's model provides a systematic approach to holistic care that integrates psychosocial and physical well-being.

Imogene King's Goal Attainment Theory

King's theory focuses on setting and achieving goals collaboratively between the nurse and client. In the context of psychosocial support, this might involve helping a client with depression establish small, measurable goals, such as participating in group therapy or practicing reality orientation techniques. The theory reinforces the importance of mutual understanding and shared decision-making in achieving positive client outcomes.

Virginia Henderson's Nature of Nursing Theory

Henderson's theory emphasizes helping clients achieve independence by addressing their basic needs, including emotional and social ones. For instance, reality orientation aligns with Henderson's principle of assisting clients in regaining autonomy by reinforcing their sense of self and connection to their environment.

4.2.2 Applying Nursing Theories to Therapeutic Interventions

The integration of these theories into psychosocial care enhances the effectiveness of therapeutic techniques by providing a structured approach to addressing client needs. For example:

- **Reminiscence Therapy**: Guided by Peplau's Interpersonal Relations Model, nurses can build trust during reminiscence sessions, allowing clients to feel comfortable sharing personal experiences.
- **Validation Therapy**: Abdellah's framework helps identify underlying emotional needs, such as fear or loneliness, that validation therapy can address.
- **Reality Orientation**: King's focus on goal setting can be applied to help clients regain orientation by establishing measurable milestones, such as recalling the day of the week or recognizing familiar faces.
- **Group Sessions**: Henderson's emphasis on independence supports the goal of group therapy to empower clients with the skills and confidence to navigate their emotional challenges collaboratively.

4.2.3 Measurable Client Outcomes

Therapeutic approaches in psychosocial support are most impactful when their outcomes can be objectively measured and evaluated. This ensures that the interventions not only address the immediate needs of the client but also contribute to long-term improvements in emotional, psychological, and social well-being. Measurable outcomes provide valuable feedback for both the nurse and the client, helping to refine therapeutic strategies and enhance the effectiveness of care.

Success in psychosocial support can manifest in various ways, depending on the chosen therapeutic approach and the client's individual goals. For example, improved client engagement is a key indicator of progress, particularly in therapies like reminiscence or group sessions, where active participation is essential. A client participating in reminiscence therapy may begin to recall and share memories more willingly, demonstrating enhanced cognitive function and emotional connectivity. Similarly, a client involved in group therapy might show increased confidence in social interactions and a stronger sense of belonging within the group, signaling reduced feelings of isolation.

Reduced anxiety is another measurable outcome that underscores the effectiveness of therapeutic interventions. Clients who engage in validation therapy, for instance, often exhibit decreased agitation or restlessness as they feel understood and validated in their experiences. Over time, this can translate into a calmer demeanor and a more positive outlook, which are critical for overall emotional resilience.

Enhanced cognitive function is particularly relevant in approaches like reality orientation, where the goal is to improve the client's ability to navigate their environment and maintain a connection to the present. A measurable outcome in this context could be the client's ability to recall the day of the week or recognize familiar faces more consistently. These small but significant milestones indicate that the therapy is effectively supporting the client's cognitive capabilities.

Emotional resilience, another important outcome, reflects a client's ability to cope with stress, adapt to challenges, and maintain a sense of purpose despite difficulties. For instance, a client who initially displays withdrawal or hopelessness may, after several sessions of therapeutic intervention, begin to express optimism about the future or actively pursue personal goals. This shift indicates a strengthened emotional foundation, enabling the client to better manage their circumstances.

For therapeutic interventions to remain effective, nurses must engage in continuous assessment and evaluation. Regularly monitoring the client's progress ensures that the chosen strategies are aligned with their evolving needs and goals. For example, if a client shows minimal progress in group therapy, the nurse might explore whether individual therapy or a different approach would be more suitable. These adjustments not only demonstrate the nurse's commitment to client-centered care but also maximize the potential for positive outcomes.

Moreover, measurable outcomes serve as a tool for fostering collaboration between the nurse and the client. When clients see tangible evidence of their progress—such as reduced symptoms of depression or improved social confidence—they are more likely to stay motivated and engaged in their therapeutic journey. This collaborative process enhances the therapeutic relationship and reinforces the client's sense of agency in their own care.

By focusing on measurable outcomes, therapeutic approaches in psychosocial support transcend abstract goals and deliver concrete, observable benefits. This not only validates the effectiveness of nursing interventions but also empowers clients to recognize and celebrate their progress, fostering a sense of achievement and hope for the future. Ultimately, these outcomes form the foundation of holistic and impactful psychosocial care, ensuring that every client receives the support they need to thrive emotionally, mentally, and socially.

4.3 Assessing Clients' Psychosocial Functioning

Assessing a client's psychosocial functioning is a critical component of nursing care, as it provides insight into their mental health, coping mechanisms, and the stressors that may influence their overall well-being. This process goes beyond observing behaviors or recording symptoms; it involves a comprehensive evaluation of the client's emotional, social, and psychological status. By understanding the client's unique experiences and challenges, nurses can develop tailored care plans that address both immediate needs and long-term goals for improved health and well-being.

One of the foundational steps in assessing psychosocial functioning is collecting accurate and detailed data about the client's coping mechanisms and the stressors affecting their care. Clients experience a wide range of stressors, including those related to their personal lives, medical conditions, and external circumstances. For instance, a client managing a chronic illness might face financial strain, family tension, or feelings of hopelessness, all of which can affect their ability to cope effectively. Nurses must engage in active listening and use open-ended questions to encourage clients to share their concerns, fears, and perspectives. This creates a clearer picture of the client's psychosocial state and helps build a trusting nurse-client relationship.

4.3.1 Psychosocial Risk Factors

Understanding psychosocial risk factors is essential for accurately assessing clients' mental health and identifying potential challenges to their care. These factors include lifestyle choices such as alcohol consumption, caffeine use, smoking, and drug abuse, all of which can significantly impact physical and emotional well-being. For example, a client with high alcohol consumption may face difficulty managing stress and may experience complications such as liver damage, emotional instability, or strained relationships. Similarly, excessive caffeine intake can exacerbate anxiety and disrupt sleep patterns, further impairing coping mechanisms.

It is also important to differentiate psychosocial risk factors from other categories such as social demographic, environmental, and biophysical factors. Social demographic factors include elements such as income level, education, and cultural background, which can shape access to care and attitudes toward health management. Environmental factors, such as living conditions or exposure to toxins, influence physical and mental health outcomes. Biophysical factors, including genetic predispositions and existing medical conditions, further complicate the psychosocial picture. By distinguishing these categories, nurses can create a multidimensional assessment that addresses all aspects of a client's health.

4.3.2 Developmental Theories in Psychosocial Assessment

Incorporating developmental theories provides nurses with a framework to understand how a client's stage of development influences their mental and emotional health. Jean Piaget's stages of cognitive development, for instance, explain how cognitive abilities evolve from infancy through adolescence, providing insights into how clients of different ages process information and make decisions. A young child in the preoperational stage may struggle with abstract concepts, while an adolescent in the formal operational stage may exhibit advanced problem-solving skills but also heightened emotional sensitivity.

Similarly, Erik Erikson's psychosocial stages of development highlight the key challenges individuals face at different life stages, such as developing trust in infancy, autonomy in early childhood, or a sense of purpose during adolescence. Understanding these stages allows nurses to tailor interventions that align with the client's developmental needs. For example, a school-aged child struggling with industry versus inferiority may benefit from encouragement and opportunities to build confidence, while an elderly client in the stage of integrity versus despair may need support in reflecting on their life and finding meaning.

Freud's psychosexual development theory adds another layer, emphasizing how early life experiences shape personality and coping mechanisms. By considering these developmental frameworks, nurses can better assess the root causes of emotional and behavioral challenges and plan interventions accordingly.

4.3.3 Recognizing and Addressing Defense Mechanisms

Defense mechanisms are unconscious strategies clients use to protect themselves from emotional distress or anxiety. Recognizing these behaviors is crucial for nurses, as they can influence the client's willingness to engage in treatment or acknowledge their condition. Common defense mechanisms include:

- **Denial**: Refusing to acknowledge a problem or its severity. For example, a client with a recent myocardial infarction may insist they are healthy and ready to resume strenuous activities.
- **Rationalization**: Justifying unacceptable behaviors or feelings with logical explanations. A client who smokes heavily might argue it helps them manage stress, minimizing its health risks.
- **Projection**: Attributing one's own unacceptable feelings or thoughts to others. A client experiencing guilt may accuse others of judging them harshly.
- **Conversion Reaction**: Transforming psychological stress into physical symptoms, such as unexplained paralysis or pain.

These mechanisms, while often unhelpful in the long term, serve as coping tools for clients in distress. Nurses must approach these behaviors with empathy, recognizing them as attempts to manage overwhelming emotions. Therapeutic communication techniques, such as reflective listening and validating the client's feelings, can help clients become more self-aware and open to addressing their challenges. For instance, when a client in denial resists discussing their condition, the nurse might gently say, "It sounds like this diagnosis feels overwhelming right now. Let's talk about how we can take it one step at a time."

4.3.4 Tailoring Interventions to Developmental and Psychosocial Needs

A comprehensive psychosocial assessment allows nurses to develop care plans that consider both the client's developmental stage and their psychosocial risk factors. For example, an adolescent with anxiety may benefit from group therapy that fosters peer support, while an older adult with depression might respond better to reminiscence therapy that helps them find meaning in their life experiences.

Practical applications of psychosocial theories in care planning include:

- Using Erikson's stages to guide age-appropriate interventions, such as promoting initiative in preschool-aged children or supporting autonomy in young adults.
- Applying Piaget's theories to tailor communication styles, ensuring that information is pre-

sented in ways that align with the client's cognitive abilities.

- Recognizing the influence of Freud's theories in addressing unresolved emotional conflicts that may manifest as behavioral or psychological symptoms.

By integrating these theories into practice, nurses can provide interventions that not only address immediate concerns but also promote long-term emotional resilience and well-being.

4.3.5 Recognizing Signs of Stress and Psychosocial Challenges

A key aspect of psychosocial assessment is identifying behaviors linked to high-risk factors, such as withdrawal, irritability, or sudden changes in mood. These signs may indicate underlying stress or ineffective coping mechanisms. For instance, a client experiencing financial stress may appear distracted, anxious, or reluctant to discuss treatment options. Recognizing these indicators allows nurses to explore the root causes of the client's distress and develop targeted interventions.

Effective strategies for managing psychosocial challenges include teaching stress management techniques, connecting clients with support networks, and fostering a therapeutic relationship that builds trust and encourages open communication. By addressing these challenges in a supportive and holistic way, nurses empower clients to navigate their circumstances with greater confidence and resilience.

4.4 Supporting Clients During Emotional or Behavioral Crises

Emotional and behavioral crises are challenging moments in healthcare that require nurses to balance empathy, vigilance, and clinical expertise. These crises, often triggered by stress, loss, trauma, or medical conditions, necessitate immediate intervention to ensure the safety and well-being of clients and caregivers. By employing effective de-escalation techniques, recognizing abnormal emotional responses, and providing tailored emotional support, nurses can help clients navigate these challenging experiences while fostering trust and resilience.

4.4.1 Recognizing and Addressing Emotional Distress

Emotional distress often manifests as anger, agitation, grief, or denial, and understanding its root causes is critical for providing effective support. Stressors such as medical uncertainty, financial strain, or feelings of helplessness can overwhelm clients, leading to heightened emotional responses. For example, a client who feels misunderstood or unheard during their care may exhibit frustration or hostility. Nurses must remain attentive to both verbal and nonverbal cues, such as raised voices, physical restlessness, or withdrawal, to identify signs of emotional distress early.

Grief and loss, in particular, require sensitive handling. Abnormal responses such as suppressed grief or prolonged denial can impede emotional healing and complicate the client's ability to engage with their care plan. Clients experiencing significant emotional trauma, such as those coping with habitual abortions, often require compassionate validation of their feelings. Simple but meaningful phrases like, "It's okay to feel this way," or, "I'm here to listen," can create a safe space for clients to express their emotions without fear of judgment. Providing resources such as counseling services or peer support groups can further help clients process their feelings and find solace in shared experiences.

4.4.2 De-Escalation Techniques and Safety Measures

In moments of heightened agitation or potential aggression, de-escalation techniques are essential to maintain a therapeutic and safe environment. These strategies are grounded in calm, empathetic communication and structured interventions that reduce tension and prevent escalation. For example, maintaining a calm tone, using open body language, and avoiding confrontational language can help diffuse a tense situation. A nurse might say, "I can see this is frustrating—let's work together to find a solution," to redirect the client's focus and foster collaboration.

Recognizing triggers for aggression is another key component of effective de-escalation. Triggers may include environmental factors such as noise or overcrowding, as well as personal stressors like fear of medical procedures or feelings of loss of control. Observing warning signs—such as clenched fists, rapid breathing, or avoidance of eye contact—allows nurses to intervene proactively. Techniques like redirecting the client's attention, providing clear choices, or acknowledging their feelings can help de-escalate situations before they become unmanageable.

Safety must remain a priority during emotional or behavioral crises. Nurses should adhere to established safety protocols, such as maintaining a safe distance, ensuring access to assistance if needed, and positioning themselves in a way that allows for easy exit if necessary. In extreme cases where de-escalation fails, involving additional team members or security personnel may be required to protect both the client and caregivers.

4.4.3 Providing Emotional Support and Promoting Resilience

Once the immediate crisis is managed, nurses must focus on supporting the client's emotional recovery. Therapeutic communication forms the foundation of this support, allowing nurses to connect with clients on a meaningful level. Active listening, reflecting emotions, and offering empathetic responses reassure clients that their experiences and feelings are valid. For instance, when a client expresses hopelessness, a nurse might respond, "It sounds like this has been really overwhelming for you. Let's talk about how we can work through this together."

Encouraging clients to express their feelings in a safe and supportive environment is critical for emotional healing. Nurses can guide clients through structured coping strategies, such as journaling, relaxation exercises, or mindfulness practices, to help them process their emotions. Referrals to counseling or therapy can further provide clients with the tools they need to develop resilience and regain a sense of control over their circumstances.

Tailoring interventions to the client's unique needs and circumstances is essential. A client dealing with grief, for example, may benefit from small, achievable goals, such as attending a support group or participating in light activities, to gradually rebuild their emotional strength. Similarly, a client managing chronic stress may find relief in techniques like guided imagery or progressive muscle relaxation, which promote calmness and focus.

4.4.4 Integrating Compassion and Clinical Expertise

Supporting clients during emotional or behavioral crises requires a balance of compassion, clinical skill, and strategic intervention. By recognizing the nuances of emotional distress, employing effective de-escalation techniques, and fostering a safe environment, nurses can guide clients through moments of intense vulnerability. Providing tailored emotional support and resources further empowers clients to process their emotions, recover their resilience, and move forward with confidence.

Through thoughtful, empathetic care, nurses play a pivotal role in not only addressing the immediate crisis but also laying the foundation for long-term emotional recovery and well-being. This holistic approach ensures that clients receive the comprehensive support they need to navigate their challenges with dignity and hope.

4.5 Providing Culturally and Spiritually Inclusive Care

Delivering culturally and spiritually inclusive care is an essential aspect of holistic nursing, ensuring that every client feels respected, valued, and understood within the healthcare environment. Culture, spirituality, gender identity, and individual preferences profoundly shape how clients experience illness, make decisions about their care, and interact with healthcare providers. Nurses, as frontline caregivers, play a pivotal role in bridging cultural gaps and creating an inclusive atmosphere where clients feel empowered to express their beliefs and values without fear of judgment or misunderstanding.

4.5.1 The Importance of Cultural Competence in Nursing

Cultural competence is the foundation of inclusive care. It involves understanding, respecting, and adapting to the diverse cultural practices, beliefs, and preferences that clients bring to their healthcare experiences. For example, a Native-American client may request the presence of a medicine woman during an examination as part of their spiritual practices. Honoring such requests not only enhances trust and client satisfaction but also underscores the nurse's commitment to respecting the client's cultural identity. Similarly, a Muslim client may have specific needs for privacy during care, such as preferring same-gender caregivers, or dietary restrictions during hospital stays. By accommodating these preferences, nurses demonstrate cultural awareness and create an environment where the client feels safe and respected.

Beyond specific examples, cultural competence requires an ongoing willingness to learn and adapt. Nurses must recognize that cultural practices are not static; they vary within communities and evolve over time. Taking the time to ask open-ended questions about a client's preferences and beliefs fosters a deeper understanding of their unique needs. For instance, a nurse might ask, "Is there anything specific about your cultural or spiritual beliefs that you would like us to consider during your care?" This not only invites dialogue but also demonstrates respect and curiosity.

4.5.2 Adapting Care Plans to Meet Cultural and Spiritual Needs

Developing culturally inclusive care plans involves integrating the client's beliefs and preferences into all aspects of their care while adhering to professional and ethical standards. This requires flexibility, empathy, and clear communication between the nurse, the client, and other members of the healthcare team. For example, when working with clients who incorporate traditional healing practices, nurses should strive to understand these methods and explore how they can complement, rather than conflict with, conventional treatments. A client using herbal remedies for a chronic condition, for instance, might benefit from a discussion about how these remedies interact with prescribed medications, ensuring safety while respecting the client's choices.

The nurse's role in facilitating culturally sensitive care extends beyond direct client interactions. Advocacy is critical, particularly when cultural needs may conflict with institutional policies or healthcare norms. For instance, a client nearing the end of life may wish to engage in specific rituals or have a spiritual advisor present. The nurse can advocate for these requests, educating other healthcare team members about their significance and coordinating the necessary accommodations. Such efforts not only respect the client's values but also model cultural competence for the broader team.

4.5.3 Practical Strategies for Integrating Cultural and Spiritual Beliefs

Integrating cultural and spiritual beliefs into care requires proactive planning and a commitment to inclusivity. Practical strategies include:

- **Accommodating Spiritual Advisors and Traditional Healers**: Nurses should facilitate access to spiritual or religious advisors when requested, whether it involves arranging visits from a chaplain, rabbi, or imam, or ensuring that a client's traditional healer is part of their care team. For example, allowing a Native-American client to participate in a smudging ceremony in a private space can significantly enhance their sense of well-being and trust in the healthcare process.
- **Honoring Dietary Practices**: Clients from various religious or cultural backgrounds often have specific dietary restrictions or preferences. Nurses can work with dietary teams to ensure that meals align with these needs, such as providing kosher meals for Jewish clients or halal options for Muslim clients.
- **Respecting Gender Identity and Expression**: Providing care that aligns with a client's gen-

der identity involves using their preferred pronouns, addressing them appropriately, and ensuring privacy and dignity during all aspects of care. For instance, offering same-gender caregivers or private changing areas may help a transgender client feel more comfortable.

- **Recognizing End-of-Life Preferences**: Cultural and spiritual beliefs often play a significant role in how clients approach end-of-life care. Nurses should explore these beliefs with sensitivity, ensuring that rituals, family involvement, and other preferences are honored whenever possible.

These strategies not only enhance the client's experience but also build trust, reduce stress, and improve outcomes by addressing the holistic dimensions of care.

4.5.4 Fostering an Inclusive and Respectful Environment

Cultural and spiritual inclusivity in nursing is about more than individual interactions; it requires creating a healthcare environment that actively promotes respect and equity. Nurses are responsible for setting the tone by modeling cultural awareness, educating colleagues about diverse practices, and addressing behaviors or policies that may unintentionally marginalize clients. For instance, correcting assumptions or stereotypes about a client's cultural background during team discussions helps foster a more inclusive culture within the healthcare setting.

Professionalism is central to this effort. Nurses must balance cultural sensitivity with clinical judgment, ensuring that care decisions reflect both respect for the client's beliefs and adherence to evidence-based practices. For example, if a traditional healing practice poses a potential risk to the client's health, the nurse should address the concern tactfully, providing education and exploring safer alternatives without dismissing the client's cultural values.

4.5.5 Enhancing Client Trust and Satisfaction

When nurses prioritize cultural and spiritual inclusivity, they create a foundation of trust that significantly enhances the client's overall experience. Clients who feel their beliefs are respected are more likely to engage in their care, adhere to treatment plans, and express their needs openly. This trust fosters stronger nurse-client relationships, ultimately contributing to better health outcomes and greater client satisfaction.

Culturally and spiritually inclusive care is an integral part of holistic nursing. By understanding and honoring the diverse values, practices, and preferences of their clients, nurses not only meet their professional obligations but also create meaningful connections that empower clients to feel valued and supported. Through active listening, thoughtful planning, and advocacy, nurses can ensure that every client receives care that respects their unique identity, fostering dignity, trust, and healing.

4.6 Addressing Noncompliance and Barriers to Care

Noncompliance with treatment plans is a multifaceted challenge that can significantly impact client outcomes. It often arises from a combination of physical, cognitive, sensory, and psychosocial factors, requiring nurses to adopt a holistic approach to care. By identifying and addressing the underlying barriers to compliance, nurses can develop strategies that promote adherence, improve recovery outcomes, and enhance the overall quality of care. This section delves into these barriers and explores practical interventions that empower clients to actively participate in their treatment.

4.6.1 Understanding Reasons for Noncompliance

Noncompliance with treatment plans is rarely a conscious decision by clients. Instead, it often results from barriers that they may be unable to recognize or overcome without support. Physical, sensory, cognitive, and emotional factors can all play a role, making it essential for nurses to identify these challenges early and develop effective interventions to address them.

Physical and Sensory Barriers

Sensory and physical impairments are among the most significant contributors to noncompliance. Conditions like **unilateral neglect**, often seen in clients recovering from strokes or brain injuries, can limit their ability to adhere to prescribed routines. A client with unilateral neglect might fail to recognize one side of their body, resulting in behaviors such as neglecting to groom or dress that side or ignoring meals placed within their blind spot. These behaviors, while unintentional, can lead to incomplete rehabilitation or inadequate self-care.

In these cases, nurses must focus on interventions that promote awareness and adaptation. For example, techniques like **placing items on the affected side to encourage attention** or using mirrors to enhance spatial awareness can help clients engage more effectively with their environment. Collaboration with occupational or physical therapists further strengthens these strategies, ensuring the client receives comprehensive support.

Other sensory challenges, such as vision or hearing loss, also hinder compliance. A client with low vision may struggle with tasks like reading medication instructions or navigating their environment safely, while those with hearing impairments might miss verbal instructions. Nurses can bridge these gaps by providing **clear, accessible communication**, such as written instructions in large print, visual aids, or assistive devices like amplified phones.

Emotional and Psychosocial Factors

Fear, anxiety, and a lack of understanding about their condition or treatment plan are common emotional barriers to compliance. For example, a client managing a chronic condition may feel overwhelmed by a complex medication schedule or unsure about the necessity of certain treatments. These emotional responses often manifest as avoidance or inconsistent adherence.

Nurses play a crucial role in addressing these concerns by fostering trust through **therapeutic communication**. Techniques like **active listening, empathy, and validation** allow clients to express their fears and frustrations, creating an open dialogue about their challenges. For instance, if a client voices concerns about side effects, a nurse can provide reassurance and education, explaining potential outcomes and offering solutions to mitigate discomfort.

Family dynamics also contribute to noncompliance. A client experiencing strained relationships or limited support at home may lack the encouragement needed to follow through with treatments. Nurses should assess the client's support system and, when necessary, involve family members in education and care planning to foster a collaborative approach to compliance.

4.6.2 Environmental Factors in Compliance

The environment in which care is delivered plays a critical role in either supporting or hindering compliance. Clients with conditions like **myasthenia gravis**, for instance, require calm and low-stress surroundings to minimize symptom exacerbations and ensure adherence to treatment plans. A quiet, well-organized space can reduce fatigue and stress, both of which are known to worsen symptoms. In shared rooms, pairing these clients with a quiet, non-disruptive roommate can greatly enhance their comfort and overall well-being. Conversely, placing them in a room with a disruptive or overly active individual may lead to heightened anxiety, reduced engagement with care, and a decline in treatment adherence.

Nurses are pivotal in assessing and tailoring the care environment to meet these needs. This involves not only selecting appropriate room placements but also identifying potential environmental triggers that might impact compliance. For example, excessive noise, poor lighting, or a lack of privacy can significantly hinder a client's recovery and engagement in their care plan. Simple interventions, such as ensuring low lighting during rest periods or providing noise-canceling options like earplugs, can make a substantial difference in the client's experience.

Practical Strategies for Optimizing Care Environments

Creating an environment that supports compliance requires intentional design and consistent effort. Strategies include:

- **Reducing Noise Levels**: Using sound-absorbing materials, maintaining quiet hours, and minimizing unnecessary interruptions in shared rooms help create a calm atmosphere.
- **Enhancing Lighting**: Ensuring adequate natural or artificial light during the day while dimming lights at night promotes better sleep and recovery.
- **Providing Restful Spaces**: Creating private areas where clients can relax or meditate can significantly reduce stress levels and improve focus on their care routines.

Nurses also have a responsibility to educate both clients and families about how the care environment influences recovery. For example, helping families understand the need for calm surroundings at home can lead to adjustments that better support the client, such as creating a designated quiet space or organizing the home to reduce physical and mental stress.

A Collaborative Approach to Environmental Compliance

Optimizing the environment is a collaborative effort between healthcare providers, clients, and their families. By involving all stakeholders in decisions about the care setting, nurses can foster a shared commitment to creating conditions that enhance compliance and recovery. Encouraging clients to voice their preferences about their environment not only empowers them but also ensures that their specific needs are met. For instance, a client may request softer lighting or prefer to have personal items nearby for comfort, which can contribute positively to their well-being.

By taking a proactive and client-centered approach, nurses ensure that environmental factors become an asset rather than a barrier to compliance. Such thoughtful adjustments not only improve adherence to treatment plans but also foster a sense of dignity, comfort, and empowerment for clients as they navigate their recovery journey.

4.6.3 Interventions for Sensory and Cognitive Impairments

Sensory and cognitive impairments require thoughtful, specialized interventions that address the unique challenges faced by clients. These impairments often hinder a client's ability to follow treatment protocols or engage in daily activities, making targeted nursing strategies essential to improving adherence and quality of life. Nurses must assess each client's specific needs and tailor interventions to promote functional recovery and independence.

In cases of **unilateral neglect**, a common condition following strokes or brain injuries, clients may fail to recognize or respond to one side of their body or environment. This can lead to behaviors such as neglecting to dress one side of the body or overlooking food on one side of their plate. To address this, nurses can implement strategies that encourage awareness of the neglected side. For example, placing commonly used items, such as utensils or grooming tools, on the affected side prompts the client to engage with that area. Additionally, nurses can guide clients through **environmental scanning exercises**, encouraging them to visually and physically explore their surroundings systematically. This practice helps to retrain the brain and improve functional awareness over time. Activities like encouraging the use of the neglected limb during simple tasks, such as holding a cup or brushing teeth, further support recovery.

For clients with **cognitive impairments**, simplifying treatment protocols is key to promoting adherence. Complex instructions can overwhelm clients with memory or processing difficulties, leading to missed medications or incomplete treatments. Breaking down instructions into smaller, more manageable steps enhances understanding and reduces the risk of errors. For instance, using a **color-coded medication organizer** paired with written instructions in clear, simple language can help clients adhere to their medication schedules. Incorporating visual aids, such as charts or infographics, provides additional clarity and reinforces learning.

Regular check-ins also play a critical role in supporting clients with cognitive impairments. These check-ins allow nurses to monitor adherence, address questions, and adjust interventions as needed. For example, scheduling brief follow-up sessions to review medication routines or demonstrate a care task helps reinforce understanding and build the client's confidence.

Supporting Independence and Building Confidence

A critical aspect of working with clients who have sensory or cognitive impairments is fostering a sense of independence and self-reliance. Encouraging clients to participate actively in their care reinforces their confidence and improves outcomes. For instance, involving clients in goal-setting can empower them to take ownership of their recovery. A nurse might work with a client to set small, achievable goals, such as using the affected limb during one meal a day or successfully managing their medications for a week. Celebrating these milestones reinforces positive behaviors and motivates clients to continue making progress.

Caregiver involvement is also essential in supporting clients with sensory or cognitive impairments. Educating family members or caregivers about the client's condition and demonstrating effective interventions ensures consistency in care. For example, caregivers can be taught to cue clients to scan their environment or assist with organizing medications. Providing caregivers with tools and strategies not only enhances the client's care but also alleviates some of the stress associated with caregiving.

4.6.4 Client Education as a Key to Compliance

Effective client education is a cornerstone of addressing noncompliance and promoting better health outcomes. Tailoring education to the client's cognitive, emotional, and physical needs ensures that information is not only understandable but also actionable. By focusing on clarity, accessibility, and practicality, nurses can empower clients to take an active role in their care and overcome barriers to adherence.

One of the most impactful strategies for improving compliance is **simplifying medication regimens**, particularly for clients managing multiple prescriptions. Consolidating medications into fewer doses or aligning administration times with the client's daily routine reduces complexity and enhances adherence. For example, a client who must take medications three times a day may benefit from adjusting doses to coincide with meals, making it easier to remember. Nurses should work closely with prescribing physicians to explore opportunities for streamlining regimens and reducing the burden of complicated schedules.

In addition to medication management, education must address the unique challenges faced by clients with **sensory impairments**. For a client with partial blindness, tactile labeling of medication bottles, such as using raised symbols or Braille, can promote independence and confidence. Similarly, arranging personal items in consistent, easily accessible locations minimizes frustration and ensures that clients can navigate their environment effectively. Nurses can demonstrate these techniques during care interactions and encourage clients to practice them until they feel comfortable.

Caregiver education is equally critical in supporting compliance, particularly for clients with **cognitive impairments**. Caregivers often play a central role in ensuring that the client follows treatment plans, so equipping them with the knowledge and skills to provide consistent support is essential. For instance, teaching caregivers to use visual aids, like medication schedules or charts, can simplify routines and reduce errors. Additionally, caregivers should be encouraged to provide gentle reminders or cues to help clients stay on track with their care plans. This collaborative approach fosters continuity of care and reinforces adherence outside the clinical setting.

Beyond these practical strategies, **building trust and rapport** through education enhances the client's confidence in their care plan. Nurses should adopt an empathetic and patient-centered approach, actively listening to the client's concerns and addressing them with sensitivity. For example, if a client expresses fear about medication side effects, a nurse might provide clear, evidence-based information about what to expect and how to manage potential issues. Offering this level of support not only alleviates anxiety but also strengthens the client's commitment to their treatment.

The Role of Repetition and Reinforcement

Education is most effective when it is delivered consistently and reinforced over time. Clients may not retain all the information provided in a single session, especially if they are overwhelmed or distracted. Nurses should incorporate repetition into their education plans, reviewing key points during subsequent visits and offering written materials for reference. Tools like pamphlets, instructional videos, or mobile apps can supplement in-person education and provide clients with ongoing support.

Additionally, feedback and follow-up are crucial to ensuring that clients and caregivers fully understand the care plan. Scheduling regular check-ins allows nurses to assess progress, address questions, and adjust strategies as needed. For example, a nurse might revisit medication routines with a client who is still struggling with adherence, offering alternative solutions like setting alarms or using pill organizers.

4.6.5 The Nurse's Role in Mitigating Barriers to Care

Nurses are uniquely positioned to identify, address, and mitigate the various barriers that can hinder a client's ability to comply with treatment plans. This requires a proactive and multifaceted approach, beginning with comprehensive assessments to uncover physical, sensory, cognitive, and emotional challenges that may impede adherence. These assessments are not one-size-fits-all; instead, they must be tailored to the client's unique circumstances to fully understand the obstacles they face.

For instance, a nurse might observe that a client struggles to retain verbal instructions due to memory impairment. In response, the nurse could provide written materials with simple, step-by-step guidance or suggest using visual aids to reinforce learning. Enlisting the support of family members or caregivers ensures continuity of care outside the clinical setting and offers additional support for clients who may otherwise feel overwhelmed.

Advocacy and Environmental Adaptations

Advocacy is a critical component of the nurse's role in overcoming barriers to care. This involves ensuring that the care environment supports recovery and addressing systemic issues that may hinder a client's ability to engage fully in their treatment. For example, language barriers can prevent clients from understanding instructions or asking questions about their care. In such cases, nurses should facilitate access to interpreters or culturally appropriate resources that enable effective communication. Similarly, clients with financial constraints may struggle to afford medications or treatments. Nurses can act as advocates by connecting clients with community resources, social services, or programs that provide financial assistance.

Nurses also play a vital role in adapting the care environment to align with the client's needs. This might involve simple changes, such as ensuring a client with sensory impairments has access to assistive devices, or more complex adjustments, like collaborating with an interdisciplinary team to develop a comprehensive care plan. For example, occupational therapists can help clients develop skills to manage physical limitations, while social workers can address psychosocial and resource-related barriers.

Collaboration with Interdisciplinary Teams

Effective care often requires the input and expertise of multiple professionals. Nurses act as coordinators within the interdisciplinary team, ensuring that all aspects of the client's care are addressed holistically. For instance, a client recovering from a stroke who struggles with both cognitive impairments and mobility challenges may benefit from a collaborative approach involving physical therapists, speech therapists, and mental health professionals. The nurse's role in this process includes advocating for the client's needs, facilitating communication among team members, and ensuring that the care plan is both cohesive and client-centered.

Collaboration also extends to involving the client and their family in the care planning process. By fostering open communication and shared decision-making, nurses empower clients to take ownership of their health. This not only enhances adherence but also builds trust and a sense of partnership in the care process.

4.6.6 Fostering Compliance Through Individualized Care

Addressing noncompliance and overcoming barriers to care requires a **client-centered approach** that prioritizes the individual needs, preferences, and circumstances of each client. By tailoring interventions to align with the unique challenges and strengths of the client, nurses can foster a sense of ownership and active participation in the care process. This personalized approach is key to creating a partnership between the client and the healthcare team, which in turn promotes adherence and improves outcomes.

A vital component of individualized care is **involving the client in the decision-making process**.

Rather than imposing changes or adjustments unilaterally, nurses should engage clients in discussions about their care plans. For example, when considering medication adjustments, explaining the rationale behind the changes and seeking the client's input can encourage collaboration and build trust. A client who feels heard and valued is more likely to commit to their treatment plan and follow through with prescribed interventions.

Empathy and Understanding: Building Bridges to Compliance

Fostering compliance is as much about addressing emotional and psychological barriers as it is about resolving logistical ones. Nurses must approach each client with empathy, seeking to understand their perspective and the factors influencing their behavior. A client who appears resistant to care may be struggling with fear, anxiety, or a lack of understanding about their condition. In such cases, taking the time to listen, validate their feelings, and provide clear, supportive education can make a significant difference.

For instance, a client with a chronic condition like diabetes may express frustration over dietary restrictions or frequent medication administration. By empathizing with these challenges and offering practical solutions—such as meal planning tips or strategies to simplify medication routines—nurses can help clients feel more in control of their care. This approach not only reduces resistance but also empowers clients to make sustainable changes that support their health.

The Holistic Impact of Individualized Care

Individualized care extends beyond addressing immediate health concerns to encompass the client's broader well-being. Nurses should consider factors such as the client's cultural background, family dynamics, and social support network when developing care plans. For example, a client from a close-knit family may benefit from involving family members in education sessions or care planning, while a client with limited social support might require referrals to community resources or support groups.

Tailoring interventions to the client's specific circumstances also demonstrates respect for their autonomy and identity. This might involve accommodating cultural practices, adapting communication styles to suit the client's preferences, or addressing language barriers to ensure understanding. By creating a care plan that reflects the client's values and priorities, nurses reinforce their role as advocates and partners in care.

4.7 Promoting Self-Esteem and Emotional Support

Fostering self-esteem and providing emotional support are foundational aspects of nursing care, directly influencing a client's emotional well-being and overall recovery. Nurses play a critical role in addressing concerns about self-image, building trust, and encouraging a positive outlook in clients across all developmental stages. By understanding the psychological and developmental needs of clients, nurses can provide tailored support that empowers individuals to navigate challenges with confidence and resilience.

To promote self-esteem effectively, it is essential for nurses to consider developmental theories, such as **Erik Erikson's stages of psychosocial development**, as a framework for understanding age-appropriate challenges. For instance, preschool-aged children are in the stage of developing initiative and a sense of purpose. They thrive when provided opportunities for exploration and positive reinforcement, which encourage their growing independence. Nurses can support these children by involving them in simple, age-appropriate tasks during care, such as choosing a bandage color or participating in pretend play that incorporates medical tools. These activities not only foster initiative but also help reduce fear associated with medical procedures.

Similarly, school-aged children are focused on developing industry and self-confidence. This stage is marked by a desire to master new skills and gain recognition for accomplishments. For these clients, nurses can promote self-esteem by providing clear instructions, setting achievable goals, and celebrating their efforts. For example, a nurse might encourage a child to keep a chart tracking their progress in physical therapy, offering praise for each milestone achieved. Such positive reinforcement builds a sense of competence and motivates continued effort.

For adults, challenges to self-esteem often center around body image, emotional resilience, and the ability to maintain their roles and responsibilities. Conditions that temporarily alter physical appearance, such as **Kawasaki disease** or injuries requiring extensive bandaging, can lead to significant anxiety and concerns about self-image. In these cases, nurses can alleviate fears by providing **clear education about disease progression and recovery timelines**, reassuring clients that changes are temporary. For instance, explaining that symptoms like skin desquamation or swelling will resolve over time and discussing how clients can care for themselves during recovery fosters trust and reduces anxiety. This information not only reassures clients but also strengthens their confidence in the care process.

Therapeutic communication is a cornerstone of promoting self-esteem and emotional support. Nurses must adopt a client-centered approach, using active listening, empathy, and validation to address emotional concerns. Validating a client's fears or frustrations, such as acknowledging the difficulty of managing a chronic condition or dealing with temporary physical changes, helps clients feel understood and supported. Clear, empathetic explanations about the care process and the rationale for specific interventions further build trust and alleviate uncertainty. For example, when a client expresses concerns about long-term scars from a procedure, a nurse can provide reassurance by discussing potential treatments for scar reduction and emphasizing the positive aspects of the recovery journey.

Practical strategies for therapeutic communication can be applied across different developmental stages. For younger clients, fostering initiative might involve engaging them in interactive activities that normalize their medical experiences, such as reading storybooks about hospital visits. For school-aged children, building industry could include involving them in age-appropriate decisions about their care, like choosing a flavor of medication. For adults, addressing self-esteem challenges might involve encouraging self-care routines or connecting them with support groups where they can share experiences with others facing similar challenges.

Education is another vital tool for promoting self-esteem and emotional resilience. Clients and families who understand the progression of a condition, the steps involved in recovery, and what to expect along the way are better equipped to manage their emotions and maintain a positive outlook. Nurses should provide information in a manner that is accessible and relevant to the client's needs, using tools such as diagrams, handouts, or demonstrations to enhance understanding. For families of children with conditions like Kawasaki disease, educating them about expected timelines for recovery and reinforcing the temporary nature of physical changes can alleviate their anxiety and help them support the child effectively.

Nurses also have a responsibility to uplift and empower clients, helping them recognize their strengths and achievements. This might involve highlighting the progress a client has made, celebrating small victories, or simply reminding them of their resilience in the face of adversity. For example, a nurse caring for a client recovering from a stroke might point out how far they've come in regaining mobility, reinforcing their ability to overcome challenges.

4.8 Substance Abuse Recognition and Intervention

Substance abuse recognition and intervention is a critical area of nursing care, requiring a deep understanding of the physical, emotional, and social dimensions of substance use disorders. Nurses play a pivotal role in identifying clients who may be struggling with substance abuse, addressing withdrawal symptoms, and providing interventions that promote recovery and well-being. This area of care demands a compassionate, nonjudgmental approach to build trust and encourage clients to engage with the care process.

Recognizing substance use disorders begins with a thorough assessment of the client's physical, behavioral, and psychological state. **Key indicators** of substance abuse may include unexplained changes in mood, erratic behavior, poor hygiene, or physical signs such as track marks, dilated or constricted pupils, and significant weight loss or gain. Clients may also exhibit frequent requests for specific medications, inconsistencies in their medical history, or unexplained injuries, all of which can signal potential substance abuse. Nurses should approach these observations with sensitivity, creating an open and safe environment for the client to disclose their concerns.

Withdrawal symptoms vary depending on the substance involved but often include physical and psychological distress. For example, clients withdrawing from alcohol may experience tremors, agitation, nausea, sweating, and even life-threatening complications like seizures or delirium tremens (DTs). Withdrawal from opioids, while less likely to be fatal, is intensely uncomfortable and marked by symptoms such as muscle aches, insomnia, diarrhea, vomiting, and severe cravings. Stimulant withdrawal often presents with fatigue, depression, and increased appetite, while withdrawal from sedatives may involve anxiety, restlessness, and rebound insomnia. Understanding these symptoms is essential for prompt recognition and intervention.

Nursing interventions during withdrawal focus on **stabilizing the client, managing symptoms, and providing supportive care**. Monitoring vital signs is a priority, as withdrawal can cause fluctuations in blood pressure, heart rate, and temperature. For example, in alcohol withdrawal, close observation for hypertension and tachycardia is essential, as these signs may indicate the onset of more severe complications. In cases of opioid withdrawal, nurses may administer medications such as methadone or buprenorphine to alleviate symptoms and reduce cravings, while benzodiazepines are often used to manage alcohol withdrawal symptoms safely.

Supportive care extends beyond physical stabilization to address the client's emotional and psychological needs. Withdrawal is often accompanied by feelings of shame, guilt, or hopelessness, which can hinder the recovery process. Nurses should employ **therapeutic communication techniques** to validate the client's experiences and provide reassurance. For example, expressing empathy and normalizing the difficulty of withdrawal can help reduce feelings of isolation and encourage the client to remain engaged in treatment.

Education is another key component of intervention, as clients must understand the importance of ongoing treatment and the risks of relapse. Nurses should provide clear, tailored information about the effects of substance use, the benefits of recovery, and available support systems. This may include discussing the role of counseling, group therapy, or medication-assisted treatment (MAT) in sustaining recovery. For instance, explaining how MAT can reduce cravings and stabilize brain chemistry may alleviate fears or misconceptions about its use.

Addressing substance abuse also requires a **multidisciplinary approach**. Nurses often collaborate with physicians, social workers, and addiction specialists to create a comprehensive care plan that meets the client's unique needs. This may involve arranging for detoxification services, connecting clients with outpatient treatment programs, or facilitating referrals to support groups like Alcoholics Anonymous (AA) or Narcotics Anonymous (NA). Nurses play a critical role in coordinating these resources, ensuring that clients have access to the tools necessary for long-term recovery.

In addition to direct client care, nurses have a responsibility to advocate for systemic changes that support individuals with substance use disorders. This includes promoting harm reduction strategies, such as providing access to naloxone for opioid overdoses or advocating for needle exchange programs to reduce the spread of infectious diseases. By addressing the broader social determinants of health that contribute to substance abuse, nurses can help create environments that support recovery and reduce stigma.

4.9 Using Therapeutic Communication and Creating a Healing Environment

Therapeutic communication and the creation of a healing environment are central to effective nursing practice. Together, they form the foundation of trust, empathy, and respect between nurses, clients, and the broader care team. By fostering a supportive and calm atmosphere, nurses can enhance client recovery, emotional well-being, and overall satisfaction with care. These principles not only guide interactions with clients but also shape the dynamics within healthcare teams, ensuring a respectful and professional environment that prioritizes client dignity and safety.

At the heart of therapeutic communication is the ability to **validate clients' feelings and decisions**. When a client expresses a choice, such as undergoing weight loss surgery, the nurse's role is to offer nonjudgmental support and empathetic understanding. For instance, responding to a client's decision with statements like, "I respect your choice and am here to support you through this journey," fosters confidence and trust. Dismissive or judgmental comments, on the other hand, can erode rapport and discourage open communication. Nurses must actively listen to clients, reflect on their concerns, and provide information in a way that empowers them to make informed decisions about their care.

Building rapport requires not only verbal skills but also **nonverbal communication techniques**. Simple actions, such as maintaining eye contact, adopting an open and attentive posture, and using appropriate touch (when culturally and contextually appropriate), convey empathy and attentiveness. These subtle cues reassure clients that their concerns are heard and valued. For example, a nurse sitting at eye level with a client during a difficult conversation demonstrates respect and a willingness to connect on a human level.

A key component of therapeutic communication is the ability to **de-escalate tension** in emotionally charged situations. Clients experiencing stress, fear, or frustration may exhibit anger or resistance. Nurses can address these emotions by staying calm, using a soft and steady tone of voice, and acknowledging the client's feelings without confrontation. For instance, saying, "I can see that this situation is really upsetting for you; let's talk about how we can make it better," diffuses tension and opens the door for collaborative problem-solving.

The therapeutic environment extends beyond individual nurse-client interactions to encompass the **broader care setting and team dynamics**. Conflicts or inappropriate interactions among healthcare team members can undermine the healing environment and negatively affect client care. Nurses must be prepared to address such situations professionally and constructively. For example, if a team member makes a dismissive remark toward a client with dementia, the nurse might privately discuss the incident with the individual, exploring the reasons behind their behavior and reinforcing the importance of respectful communication. Using clarification and constructive feedback, the nurse can foster a more cohesive and compassionate team dynamic.

In cases where client dignity and emotional well-being are at risk, the nurse's role as an advocate becomes paramount. This might involve intervening when a colleague's behavior compromises the therapeutic environment or advocating for changes to care protocols that better align with client needs. For example, ensuring that a client with dementia is treated with patience and respect during care tasks not only protects their dignity but also promotes a sense of safety and trust.

Creating a healing environment also involves **recognizing and mitigating environmental stressors**. Noise, overcrowding, and lack of privacy can exacerbate client anxiety and hinder recovery. Nurses can take steps to reduce these stressors by ensuring a quiet and comfortable setting, providing private spaces for sensitive discussions, and addressing the client's sensory preferences. For example, dimming lights and minimizing background noise during an end-of-life conversation can create a more serene and supportive atmosphere.

Therapeutic communication is particularly vital in situations where clients feel vulnerable or uncertain, such as receiving a new diagnosis or facing life-altering decisions. In these moments, clear and supportive communication is essential to promoting emotional resilience. Providing accurate information, answering questions with patience, and validating the client's emotions help alleviate fear and build confidence. For instance, explaining the steps of a medical procedure in straightforward terms while acknowledging the client's concerns creates a sense of control and preparedness.

Collaboration and conflict resolution are integral to maintaining a therapeutic environment within the care team. Nurses must be skilled in addressing misunderstandings or disagreements among colleagues, ensuring that these conflicts do not compromise client care. This requires open communication, active listening, and a commitment to finding mutually beneficial solutions. For example, if two team members disagree on a care plan, the nurse might facilitate a discussion to clarify roles and responsibilities, keeping the client's best interests at the forefront.

By combining effective communication, empathy, and a commitment to professionalism, nurses can create a therapeutic environment that prioritizes client dignity, emotional well-being, and recovery. These efforts not only enhance client outcomes but also contribute to a culture of respect and collaboration within the healthcare team. Whether addressing client concerns, supporting team dynamics, or mitigating environmental stressors, the nurse's role in fostering a healing environment is essential to the delivery of high-quality, compassionate care.

Chapter 5
Basic Care and Comfort

Chapter 5 focuses on the essential nursing interventions that form the foundation of client-centered care, emphasizing comfort, dignity, and overall well-being. These core skills address fundamental needs such as mobility, nutrition, pain management, and rest, while fostering a supportive and safe environment for clients across diverse care settings.

Through a blend of practical techniques and compassionate care, this chapter highlights the nurse's role in promoting independence, preventing complications, and enhancing the quality of life for clients. By mastering these basic yet critical aspects of nursing care, you'll be equipped to provide effective, holistic support that meets the physical and emotional needs of those in your care.

5.1 Managing Bowel and Bladder Care

Effective bowel and bladder management is a cornerstone of nursing care, playing a critical role in maintaining client comfort, dignity, and overall health. Addressing these needs requires a combination of practical skills, personalized interventions, and a compassionate approach to ensure that clients feel supported and respected during often sensitive procedures.

Bowel and bladder training programs are a vital component of care for clients experiencing incontinence, retention, or other elimination challenges. These programs are tailored to each client's specific needs, taking into account factors such as mobility, cognitive status, and the underlying cause of their condition. For instance, clients with neurogenic bladder resulting from spinal cord injuries may benefit from scheduled voiding programs or intermittent catheterization to manage retention effectively. Similarly, clients with bowel dysfunction might be supported through dietary modifications, scheduled toileting routines, and, when necessary, the use of stool softeners or suppositories to promote regularity and reduce discomfort.

Education plays a key role in the success of these programs. Nurses must provide clients and caregivers with clear, accessible information about the goals and methods of bowel and bladder training. For example, explaining the importance of hydration and high-fiber diets can empower clients to take an active role in managing their bowel health. Additionally, encouraging adherence to a consistent toileting schedule can help clients regain a sense of control and reduce the risk of accidents or complications.

Catheter care is another integral aspect of bowel and bladder management, particularly for clients with urinary retention or those recovering from surgery. Proper catheter care not only ensures client comfort but also prevents complications such as urinary tract infections (UTIs). Nurses must adhere to strict hygiene protocols when inserting or maintaining catheters, including hand hygiene, the use of sterile techniques, and regular inspection of the catheter site for signs of irritation or infection.

Bladder irrigation is a specific procedure used to flush out the bladder, often indicated for clients with blockages, blood clots, or post-surgical needs. This intervention requires precision and attentiveness to client comfort. Before initiating bladder irrigation, nurses should explain the procedure to the client, addressing any concerns and ensuring informed consent. During the procedure, monitoring the client's response is crucial, as discomfort, cramping, or resistance may indicate complications that require immediate attention.

Client comfort should always be at the forefront of bladder and bowel care interventions. This includes creating a private and respectful environment during procedures, using therapeutic communication to alleviate embarrassment or anxiety, and addressing pain or discomfort promptly. For example, ensuring proper catheter placement and minimizing tension on the tubing can prevent unnecessary discomfort and promote better outcomes.

In addition to direct interventions, nurses must remain vigilant for signs of complications related to bowel and bladder care. Early recognition of symptoms such as cloudy or foul-smelling urine, fever, or abdominal pain can indicate potential infections or other issues that require intervention. Similarly, in clients with bowel management challenges, monitoring for signs of constipation or fecal impaction is essential to prevent further complications.

Holistic care also involves supporting the emotional well-being of clients dealing with bowel and bladder issues, as these challenges can significantly impact self-esteem and quality of life. Nurses should adopt a compassionate and nonjudgmental approach, reassuring clients that these issues are common and manageable. Encouraging open communication about any concerns or discomfort can help foster trust and collaboration, ultimately improving adherence to care plans and overall outcomes.

5.2 Enhancing Mobility and Preventing Complications

Promoting mobility and preventing the complications of immobility are critical aspects of nursing care that directly impact client recovery, independence, and overall well-being. Immobility, whether temporary or long-term, can lead to a cascade of physical and psychological complications, making proactive interventions essential for preserving health and enhancing quality of life.

One of the primary goals of mobility-focused care is to maintain or restore the client's ability to move as independently as possible. This begins with a thorough assessment of the client's physical condition, including muscle strength, joint flexibility, balance, and endurance. Based on this evaluation, nurses can develop tailored mobility plans that align with the client's capabilities and goals. For instance, a client recovering from surgery may benefit from gradually increasing their level of activity through supervised ambulation or physical therapy, while a client with paralysis may require assistive devices such as wheelchairs or transfer boards to maintain functional mobility.

In clients who are unable to mobilize independently, preventing complications of immobility becomes a top priority. **Deep vein thrombosis (DVT)** is a common and potentially life-threatening complication that can occur due to prolonged immobility. Nurses play a critical role in reducing this risk through interventions such as encouraging regular movement, performing passive range-of-motion (ROM) exercises, and applying compression devices or stockings as prescribed. Additionally, educating clients about the importance of hydration and periodic leg movements can empower them to actively participate in DVT prevention.

Contractures, another significant complication, result from prolonged immobility and the shortening of muscles and tendons around joints. Preventing contractures involves consistent positioning, regular ROM exercises, and the use of splints or braces when appropriate. For example, a nurse might assist a client with stretching exercises to maintain joint flexibility or position pillows strategically to prevent contractures in the elbows or knees. Early intervention is key to preserving function and preventing permanent deformities.

Maintaining or improving **skin integrity** is equally vital for immobilized clients, as prolonged pressure on certain areas of the body can lead to pressure ulcers. These injuries, often seen on bony prominences such as the sacrum, heels, and elbows, can develop quickly and become difficult to treat if not addressed early. Nurses can reduce the risk of pressure ulcers by implementing regular repositioning schedules, typically every two hours, to redistribute pressure and improve circulation. For clients using wheelchairs, providing pressure-relieving cushions and educating them on frequent weight shifts can also be beneficial.

Another critical measure for skin integrity is ensuring proper hygiene and moisture management. Excessive moisture from perspiration, incontinence, or wound drainage can weaken the skin's barrier, increasing the risk of breakdown. Nurses should promptly address these issues by cleaning and drying the affected areas, using barrier creams or moisture-wicking materials to protect the skin. Additionally, assessing the client's nutritional status is essential, as adequate protein and hydration are necessary for maintaining skin health and promoting healing.

Beyond physical interventions, **encouraging client engagement and emotional support** are integral to mobility care. Immobility can lead to feelings of helplessness, frustration, and isolation, which may further hinder recovery. Nurses should use therapeutic communication to motivate clients, celebrate progress, and set achievable goals that foster a sense of accomplishment. For example, a nurse might encourage a post-surgical client to take a few steps each day, gradually increasing their activity level and celebrating each milestone.

Creating a safe environment is another important aspect of mobility promotion. Removing trip hazards, providing assistive devices like walkers or grab bars, and ensuring adequate lighting are all steps that enhance client safety and confidence. Nurses should also educate clients and caregivers on the proper use of mobility aids to prevent falls and injuries.

Preventing complications of immobility and enhancing mobility requires a holistic and proactive approach. By combining evidence-based interventions with empathy and individualized care, nurses can significantly improve client outcomes. These efforts not only reduce the physical risks associated with immobility but also enhance clients' emotional well-being, independence, and quality of life.

5.3 Supporting Clients with Sensory Impairments

Providing effective care for clients with sensory impairments, such as visual or hearing impairments, requires a thoughtful and holistic approach that prioritizes safety, communication, and independence. Sensory impairments can affect a client's ability to interact with their environment, navigate daily activities, and communicate effectively, making it essential for nurses to address these challenges with tailored strategies and a compassionate mindset.

5.3.1 Safety First: Creating a Supportive Environment

Ensuring the safety of clients with sensory impairments is paramount, as their reduced ability to perceive environmental cues can significantly increase the risk of accidents and injuries. A supportive environment not only minimizes these risks but also fosters confidence and independence, enabling clients to navigate their surroundings with greater ease and security. For nurses, this means taking a proactive and thoughtful approach to identifying hazards, implementing modifications, and educating clients about maintaining safety in their daily lives.

For clients with **visual impairments**, a comprehensive environmental assessment is a crucial first step. Common hazards such as cluttered walkways, uneven flooring, or poorly lit areas can present significant challenges. Nurses can mitigate these risks by ensuring that pathways are clear of obstructions, organizing spaces consistently, and improving lighting to enhance visibility. For instance, adding nightlights in hallways and bathrooms can help clients feel more secure during nighttime movements. The strategic use of **contrasting colors** can also aid navigation; for example, painting doorframes or handrails in bold, contrasting shades helps clients distinguish important objects or areas. Similarly, tactile markers, such as raised dots on stair rails or textured floor indicators, provide additional cues that guide clients safely through their environment.

In settings where clients are learning to adjust to vision loss, nurses should also emphasize the importance of orientation strategies. Teaching clients to systematically scan their environment, use their hands to identify objects, and rely on landmarks can enhance their ability to navigate unfamiliar spaces. These skills, combined with environmental modifications, empower clients to maintain a sense of control and independence.

For clients with **hearing impairments**, safety measures often focus on incorporating **visual and tactile alerts** into their surroundings. Traditional auditory signals, such as fire alarms, doorbells, or phone notifications, may not be effective for these clients. Replacing or supplementing these cues with visual alarms that flash brightly or tactile alarms that vibrate can ensure that clients remain aware of their environment and any potential dangers. For example, a fire alarm system with both flashing lights and vibrations can effectively alert clients with hearing impairments to evacuate during emergencies.

Communication of safety protocols is another essential aspect of creating a supportive environment for clients with hearing impairments. Nurses must provide instructions in ways that align with the client's preferred communication method. Written materials, visual aids, or digital displays can supplement verbal explanations, ensuring that all necessary information is clearly conveyed. For clients who lip-read, maintaining face-to-face communication in well-lit areas helps facilitate understanding.

Educating clients and their families about environmental safety is an integral part of the nurse's role. Clients may need guidance on how to organize their living spaces to minimize risks. For instance, recommending that frequently used items be placed within easy reach and that furniture arrangements remain consistent can prevent confusion and accidental injuries. Families and caregivers should also be trained to support the client's safety needs without undermining their autonomy. This includes respecting the client's ability to navigate independently while being available to assist when necessary.

Beyond the immediate physical environment, nurses should consider the **broader context of safety** for clients with sensory impairments. In public spaces, clients may face additional challenges, such as navigating busy streets or crowded areas. Nurses can educate clients about assistive tools like canes, guide dogs, or personal alert devices that enhance safety outside the home. For example, teaching a visually impaired client to use a white cane not only improves navigation but also signals to others that the client may require additional space or assistance.

Creating a supportive environment extends to emotional safety as well. Sensory impairments can make clients feel vulnerable or dependent, which may lead to frustration or anxiety. Nurses should use empathetic communication to reassure clients and involve them in decisions about their care and environment. For instance, asking clients for input on room arrangements or safety adaptations ensures that the solutions are practical and aligned with their preferences, fostering a sense of agency and confidence.

5.3.2 Enhancing Communication

Communication is a cornerstone of nursing care, and for clients with sensory impairments, adapting communication methods is key to building trust, fostering collaboration, and ensuring that their needs are effectively met. Sensory impairments can present unique barriers to understanding, but with thoughtful strategies and a patient-centered approach, nurses can create meaningful and clear interactions that enhance both the care experience and client outcomes.

For clients with **visual impairments**, verbal communication takes on heightened importance. Nurses should prioritize the use of clear, descriptive language when providing instructions or orienting clients to their environment. For example, instead of vaguely stating, "Your water is here," a nurse might say, "Your water is on the table to your right, next to your plate." Such precision allows clients to visualize their surroundings and act with greater independence. Additionally, tactile guidance can complement verbal cues, particularly for tasks requiring physical interaction with objects. Placing the client's hand directly on an object or gently guiding them through a motion, such as locating a call button, reinforces understanding and fosters a sense of control.

For clients with **hearing impairments**, communication adjustments should align with their individual preferences and abilities. This may involve written communication, sign language, or assistive devices like hearing aids or amplifiers. Written notes or visual aids can be especially helpful for conveying detailed or complex information, such as medication schedules or procedural steps. For clients who use sign language, arranging for an interpreter ensures that they can fully participate in conversations about their care. Nurses should also be prepared to learn and use basic sign language phrases to facilitate communication in the absence of an interpreter, demonstrating respect and a commitment to the client's needs.

Maintaining **face-to-face communication** is critical when interacting with clients who rely on lip reading or visual cues to understand speech. Nurses should position themselves at the client's eye level in a well-lit environment, ensuring that their face is fully visible. Speaking clearly, at a moderate pace, and enunciating without exaggerating lip movements can greatly enhance comprehension. Avoiding habits like chewing gum, covering the mouth, or turning away while speaking ensures that visual cues remain accessible to the client.

Beyond verbal and visual methods, **technology and assistive tools** can play a significant role in enhancing communication. Hearing amplifiers, text-to-speech devices, and captioned telephones are just a few examples of tools that can bridge communication gaps. Nurses should familiarize themselves with these resources and educate clients on their proper use, empowering them to leverage technology to maintain effective communication in various settings.

Empathy and **active listening** are essential components of enhancing communication with clients who have sensory impairments. Nurses should create opportunities for clients to express their concerns or preferences, using open-ended questions to encourage dialogue. For instance, asking, "What's the best way for me to explain this to you?" not only helps the nurse tailor their approach but also shows respect for the client's individuality and autonomy.

Building trust through communication also involves **acknowledging and validating challenges**. Clients with sensory impairments may experience frustration or feelings of isolation when communication is difficult. Nurses can address these emotions by offering reassurance and demonstrating patience. For example, if a client with hearing loss struggles to understand instructions, the nurse might calmly repeat the information using a different approach, such as writing it down or using a visual aid, while affirming the client's efforts with a statement like, "Let's take our time with this together."

Nurses should also extend communication strategies to include **educating families and caregivers**. Teaching family members how to communicate effectively with clients who have sensory impairments fosters continuity of care and strengthens support systems. For instance, guiding family members to use descriptive language or visual aids ensures that the client's needs are consistently met in various contexts.

5.3.3 Promoting Independence

Encouraging independence in clients with sensory impairments is a fundamental aspect of nursing care, as it not only fosters confidence but also significantly enhances their overall quality of life. Sensory impairments, while presenting unique challenges, do not have to limit an individual's ability to lead a fulfilling and autonomous life. With the right support, resources, and education, clients can develop strategies to navigate their environments and manage their daily activities effectively.

For clients with **visual impairments**, independence begins with equipping them with the tools and skills they need to safely and confidently interact with their surroundings. Nurses can introduce assistive devices such as **white canes**, which are widely recognized as symbols of visual impairment and serve as invaluable tools for orientation and mobility. Training clients in the use of these devices, often in collaboration with orientation and mobility specialists, enables them to navigate their environments with greater confidence and precision. Providing additional resources, such as **large-print materials** for reading or **audio-enabled devices**, can further enhance their ability to perform daily tasks. For instance, talking thermometers, medication dispensers, or even mobile apps that provide voice-guided instructions allow clients to maintain independence in managing their health and daily routines.

Incorporating **organizational strategies** into care plans is another practical way to empower clients with visual impairments. Nurses can guide clients to arrange personal items in consistent, easily accessible locations and label them using tactile markers or Braille. These small yet effective adjustments help clients manage their environment more efficiently and reduce frustration.

For clients with **hearing impairments**, independence often hinges on the availability and proper use of **assistive technologies**. Captioning devices for televisions, vibrating alarm clocks, and amplified phones are just a few examples of tools that can bridge communication gaps and facilitate daily living. Nurses play a pivotal role in educating clients on the use of these devices, ensuring they feel comfortable integrating them into their routines. For example, demonstrating how to set up a captioning device or adjust the settings on a vibrating alarm clock can instill confidence and encourage regular use.

Empowering clients with hearing impairments also involves teaching effective communication strategies. Clients can be encouraged to advocate for themselves by informing others of their communication preferences, such as speaking face-to-face, maintaining eye contact, or using written communication when necessary. These self-advocacy skills enhance the client's ability to participate actively in social and professional settings, fostering a sense of control and agency.

Collaboration with **occupational therapists or other specialists** is another critical component of promoting independence. These professionals can provide specialized training and adaptive techniques tailored to the client's specific needs. For instance, an occupational therapist might teach a visually impaired client to prepare meals safely or help a client with hearing impairments develop strategies for managing communication in noisy environments. Nurses can coordinate these services, ensuring that clients receive comprehensive support that aligns with their goals.

Beyond practical tools and strategies, fostering independence involves addressing the emotional and psychological aspects of sensory impairments. Clients may initially feel overwhelmed or discouraged by the limitations imposed by their condition. Nurses should provide emotional support and encouragement, celebrating small achievements and reinforcing the client's progress. For example, acknowledging milestones such as successfully navigating a new environment or mastering an assistive device can boost the client's confidence and motivate further growth.

Education extends to **family members and caregivers**, who play a vital role in supporting the client's independence. Nurses can train families on how to provide assistance without fostering dependency, emphasizing the importance of allowing the client to complete tasks independently whenever possible. For example, a caregiver might be taught to provide guidance only when asked or to assist in setting up tools that the client can then use autonomously.

5.4 Addressing Pain and Comfort

Pain management is a fundamental aspect of nursing care, as unmanaged pain can significantly impact a client's physical, emotional, and psychological well-being. While pharmacological interventions are often the cornerstone of pain relief, nonpharmacological methods play a vital role in providing comprehensive and holistic care. Nurses are uniquely positioned to address pain and comfort through a combination of evidence-based practices, therapeutic communication, and individualized interventions.

Nonpharmacological pain relief methods offer effective strategies for managing pain without the use of medications, making them particularly valuable for clients who may not tolerate pharmacological treatments or who require complementary approaches to enhance comfort. **Heat therapy**, for instance, is a simple yet powerful tool for alleviating muscle tension, improving circulation, and reducing discomfort. Applying a warm compress or heating pad to the affected area can help relax muscles and relieve pain caused by conditions such as arthritis, back strain, or menstrual cramps. Nurses must ensure that heat is applied safely, monitoring the client's skin for signs of irritation or burns and adjusting the duration and temperature as needed.

Relaxation techniques are another critical component of nonpharmacological pain management. Guided imagery, deep breathing exercises, and progressive muscle relaxation can help clients focus their attention away from pain and reduce stress levels, which are often closely linked to the perception of pain. For example, teaching a client to visualize a calming environment or engage in rhythmic breathing can empower them to take an active role in managing their pain. These techniques are particularly effective for clients experiencing chronic pain or anxiety-related discomfort, as they promote a sense of control and emotional well-being.

Repositioning is an essential yet often overlooked intervention for enhancing comfort and preventing pain in clients with limited mobility. Regularly changing a client's position not only alleviates pressure on specific areas but also improves circulation and reduces the risk of pressure ulcers. For instance, turning an immobilized client every two hours or using supportive devices such as pillows or foam wedges can prevent discomfort and promote healing. Nurses should assess the client's preferences and physical condition when implementing repositioning strategies, ensuring that the interventions are both effective and respectful of the client's needs.

An equally important aspect of addressing pain and comfort is the use of **standardized pain assessment tools**, which allow nurses to evaluate and document pain levels consistently and accurately. Tools such as the Numeric Rating Scale (NRS), Wong-Baker FACES Pain Rating Scale, and Visual Analog Scale (VAS) provide clear frameworks for assessing pain intensity, enabling nurses to tailor interventions to the client's specific experience. For clients who have difficulty verbalizing their pain, such as those with cognitive impairments or language barriers, behavioral pain assessment tools like the FLACC scale (Face, Legs, Activity, Cry, Consolability) can help identify signs of discomfort based on observable behaviors.

Effective pain assessment goes beyond measuring intensity; it also involves exploring the **qualitative aspects of pain**, such as its location, duration, and characteristics. By asking clients open-ended questions like, "Can you describe what your pain feels like?" or "What makes your pain better or worse?" nurses can gain valuable insights into the underlying causes and potential triggers of pain. This information is critical for developing a personalized pain management plan that addresses the client's unique needs and preferences.

Therapeutic communication is integral to addressing pain and comfort, as it fosters trust and encourages clients to share their concerns openly. Nurses should validate the client's experience, acknowledging their pain without judgment or minimizing their feelings. Statements such as, "I understand that you're in pain, and I'm here to help," demonstrate empathy and build rapport, ensuring that the client feels supported and understood. Providing clear explanations of pain management options and involving the client in decision-making further enhances their sense of control and confidence in the care process.

Additionally, nurses play a key role in educating clients and their families about pain management strategies, empowering them to take an active role in achieving comfort. For example, teaching a client how to use a heating pad safely or guiding them through relaxation exercises equips them with practical tools they can use independently. Family members can also be involved in supporting the client's comfort, such as assisting with repositioning or creating a calming environment at home.

5.5 Nutrition and Enteral Care

Nutrition is a cornerstone of recovery and overall health, and for clients with enteral tubes, the provision of adequate nutrition requires specialized care and meticulous attention to detail. Enteral feeding is often necessary for clients who cannot meet their nutritional needs through oral intake due to conditions such as dysphagia, neurological impairments, or gastrointestinal disorders. Nurses play a vital role in ensuring that clients with enteral tubes receive the nutrients they need while maintaining their comfort, dignity, and safety.

Feeding techniques for clients with enteral tubes must be precise and tailored to the individual's needs. Whether the feeding method involves bolus, intermittent, or continuous administration, nurses must ensure that the process is conducted efficiently and without complications. Proper tube placement verification is a critical step before initiating feeding, as improper placement can lead to serious complications such as aspiration or infection. This is typically done through pH testing of gastric aspirates or, in some cases, radiographic confirmation. Regular checks of tube patency are also essential to prevent blockages and ensure that nutrients are delivered effectively.

Troubleshooting common issues with enteral tubes is another key responsibility. Blockages, for example, can occur if formula is not adequately flushed from the tube, and nurses must be prepared to address these situations promptly. Using warm water to flush the tube or, in more persistent cases, an enzymatic solution, can help resolve obstructions. Additionally, clients may experience gastrointestinal discomfort, such as bloating, nausea, or diarrhea, due to the formula's composition or feeding rate. In such cases, nurses should collaborate with dietitians to adjust the formula or feeding schedule to improve tolerance and ensure that the client's nutritional needs continue to be met.

Site care is equally important in maintaining the health and comfort of clients with enteral tubes. The area around the tube insertion site is susceptible to irritation, infection, and skin breakdown, making meticulous hygiene practices essential. Nurses should clean the site daily with warm water and mild soap, taking care to remove any debris or crusting. Drying the area thoroughly and applying barrier creams as needed can prevent irritation and promote healing. For clients with percutaneous endoscopic gastrostomy (PEG) tubes, monitoring for signs of infection, such as redness, swelling, or discharge, is critical, and any abnormalities should be reported immediately to the healthcare team.

Ensuring that clients receive adequate nutrition through their enteral feedings is a fundamental goal. This involves not only delivering the prescribed formula but also monitoring for signs that the client's nutritional needs are being met. Indicators of adequate nutrition include stable weight, improved energy levels, and normal laboratory values for markers such as albumin and electrolytes. Nurses should work closely with dietitians to assess and adjust the nutritional plan as needed, ensuring that the client receives the appropriate caloric intake and nutrient balance to support recovery and overall health.

Maintaining hygiene throughout the feeding process is paramount to preventing complications such as infections or aspiration pneumonia. Nurses should adhere to strict infection control practices, including hand hygiene and the use of gloves when handling enteral equipment. All feeding equipment, such as syringes and feeding bags, must be cleaned and replaced according to facility guidelines to minimize the risk of contamination.

Education is another critical component of enteral care, especially for clients and caregivers who may need to manage feedings at home. Nurses should provide clear, step-by-step instructions on feeding techniques, site care, and troubleshooting common issues. For example, teaching a caregiver how to recognize and address tube blockages or how to clean the insertion site effectively empowers them to provide safe and competent care. Written materials and demonstrations can reinforce learning, and nurses should encourage questions to ensure understanding.

In addition to the technical aspects of enteral care, nurses should remain attentive **to the emotional well-being** of clients. For many individuals, reliance on enteral feeding can be a challenging adjustment, both physically and emotionally. Clients may feel self-conscious about their appearance or experience a sense of loss over their ability to eat normally. Nurses can provide emotional support by validating these feelings, offering reassurance, and promoting a positive outlook. Encouraging clients to focus on the benefits of enteral feeding, such as improved energy and recovery, can help them adapt to their new circumstances.

Ultimately, enteral care involves a delicate balance of technical expertise, meticulous attention to hygiene, and compassionate client-centered care. By focusing on both the physical and emotional aspects of enteral feeding, nurses ensure that clients receive not only the nutrients they need but also the support necessary to thrive. This holistic approach enhances client outcomes, fosters independence, and underscores the vital role of nutrition in the healing process.

5.6 Providing End-of-Life Care

End-of-life care is a profound aspect of nursing practice, requiring sensitivity, compassion, and a deep commitment to preserving the dignity of clients and their families during one of life's most challenging moments. Nurses play a vital role in ensuring that clients receive holistic and respectful care in their final stages, addressing not only physical needs but also emotional, spiritual, and social aspects of the experience. Providing end-of-life care is as much about offering comfort and understanding as it is about managing clinical responsibilities.

A cornerstone of end-of-life care is **postmortem care**, which ensures that the client is treated with dignity and respect after death. This process begins with confirming the client's passing in accordance with institutional protocols and addressing any immediate needs of the family. Postmortem care involves preparing the body, which includes cleaning and positioning it in a natural, peaceful manner. This may include closing the client's eyes, gently positioning their hands, and ensuring that the environment reflects a sense of calm and reverence. Nurses must handle the body with care and professionalism, recognizing its importance to the grieving family and their memories of their loved one.

When providing postmortem care, nurses should also be mindful of the family's **cultural and spiritual practices**. Different traditions may have specific rituals or requirements for handling the body, and it is essential to honor these preferences whenever possible. For instance, some families may request a moment of prayer, the presence of a spiritual leader, or particular steps in preparing the body. Engaging with the family and asking about their wishes ensures that care aligns with their values and beliefs, fostering a sense of respect and inclusion during a deeply personal time.

In addition to the physical aspects of care, nurses must provide **emotional support and communication** to families experiencing loss. Grief manifests differently for each person, ranging from intense sadness to disbelief or anger. Nurses should approach these emotions with empathy and patience, offering a listening ear and validating the family's feelings. Simple statements such as, "I'm here if you need someone to talk to," or "It's okay to feel what you're feeling right now," can provide immense comfort. Avoiding clichés or dismissive phrases is crucial, as they can unintentionally minimize the depth of the family's loss.

Clear and compassionate communication is also essential when discussing the client's condition during the dying process. Families often have questions about what to expect or may seek reassurance that their loved one is comfortable. Nurses should provide honest yet gentle explanations, addressing concerns about pain management or physical changes that may occur. For example, explaining that certain signs, such as labored breathing or changes in skin color, are a natural part of the dying process can help alleviate fear and uncertainty.

Supporting the family's emotional needs also extends to creating an environment where they feel welcome and involved. Allowing family members to spend time with their loved one, participate in care activities, or simply hold their hand can provide a sense of connection and closure. For families who wish to be present at the time of death, nurses should respect their choice and offer guidance on how to be there in a meaningful and comforting way.

End-of-life care often includes addressing the client's and family's **spiritual needs**, which can be a significant source of comfort during this time. Nurses can facilitate access to spiritual advisors, chaplains, or other support resources, regardless of the family's faith or belief system. Offering these services without assumption or judgment ensures that the care provided is inclusive and respectful of diverse perspectives.

While supporting the family is a primary focus, nurses must also consider their own emotional well-being when providing end-of-life care. Witnessing the death of a client and supporting grieving families can be emotionally taxing. Nurses should seek support from colleagues, supervisors, or professional counseling services to process their experiences and maintain their own mental health. Reflecting on the meaningful impact of their role in a client's final moments can also provide a sense of fulfillment and purpose.

Chapter 6
Pharmacological Therapies

Pharmacological therapies are integral to nursing practice, requiring accuracy, knowledge, and attention to detail to ensure client safety and effective care. This chapter provides essential guidance on administering medications, educating clients, and evaluating treatment outcomes. By addressing key principles such as dosage calculations, administration techniques, and medication safety, it prepares nurses to handle a wide range of pharmacological needs with confidence.

Throughout the chapter, practical strategies, real-world examples, and evidence-based interventions are emphasized to enhance understanding. Topics include medication safety, client education, pain management, and the use of specialized devices, all tailored to equip nurses with the skills needed for safe and effective pharmacological care in various clinical settings.

6.1 Performing Calculations and Medication Administration Basics

Accurate medication calculations are vital to ensure safe and effective pharmacological therapies. This section breaks down the fundamental aspects of medication calculations into two key areas: **Unit Conversions and Real-World Applications** and **Steps for Performing Accurate Calculations and Error Prevention**. By mastering these skills, nurses can confidently administer medications across diverse clinical settings.

6.1.1 Unit Conversions and Real-World Applications

Unit conversions are the cornerstone of accurate medication administration and are fundamental to ensuring safe and effective pharmacological care. Nurses must be adept at converting measurements between units such as minims, milliliters, fluid ounces, and drops, as these are commonly encountered in clinical practice. This skill is not merely theoretical; it directly impacts client safety and treatment outcomes. For instance, understanding that 1 minim equals approximately 0.06 milliliters or that 1 ounce equals 30 milliliters is vital when converting prescriptions into actionable doses. Accurate conversions can prevent errors that might otherwise lead to underdosing, overdosing, or delays in care.

Consider a scenario where a physician orders 1 milliliter of a liquid medication, but the packaging specifies dosages in minims. To administer the correct dose, the nurse must calculate the equivalent 16 minims. Similarly, in intravenous (IV) therapy, calculating flow rates often involves converting milliliters per hour into drops per minute. This requires a clear understanding of the drop factor (e.g., 15 drops per milliliter or 60 drops per milliliter, depending on the tubing used) to ensure the IV delivers the correct amount of fluid or medication over a specified time. These situations highlight the practical importance of mastering unit conversions to provide timely and accurate care.

To prepare for real-world application and the NCLEX-PN exam, it's helpful to practice common calculations. For example:

- Converting a 0.5-ounce order into milliliters: Multiply 0.5 by 30 to get 15 milliliters.
- Determining the number of minims in 2 milliliters: Multiply 2 by 16 to get 32 minims.
- Calculating an IV flow rate: If the order is for 125 milliliters per hour using tubing with a drop factor of 20 drops per milliliter, the calculation would be 125×20/60 = 41.7125 drops per minute, rounded to 42 drops per minute.

These calculations reinforce the relationship between theoretical knowledge and clinical practice, ensuring that nurses are prepared to handle diverse and complex scenarios. Understanding unit conversions also supports error prevention, a critical focus in pharmacological care. For instance, decimal placement errors can result in administering a dose ten times larger or smaller than intended. Such mistakes are easily avoidable with careful attention to detail and a strong grasp of conversion principles.

In addition to routine practice, developing strategies for quick verification during exams and in clinical settings is essential. Double-checking calculations, using trusted references, and employing systematic approaches (such as the "dimensional analysis" method) are effective ways to ensure accuracy. Dimensional analysis, in particular, is a step-by-step process that aligns units across a calculation to arrive at the correct dose systematically. For example, when converting a prescription written as 500 milligrams to its equivalent volume in milliliters based on a concentration of 250 milligrams per 5 milliliters, the calculation would proceed as follows:

$$500 \text{ mg} \times \frac{5 \text{ mL}}{250 \text{ mg}} = 10 \text{ mL}$$

This systematic approach reduces the likelihood of errors and builds confidence in performing complex calculations.

6.1.2 Steps for Performing Accurate Calculations and Error Prevention

Medication calculations are a critical skill for nurses, requiring a systematic approach to ensure safety and precision in administration. By following a clear, step-by-step process, nurses can confidently handle even complex scenarios, reducing the likelihood of errors and ensuring optimal client outcomes.

Step-by-Step Calculation Process

1. Understand the Formula:

Begin with a standard formula, such as:

$$\text{Dose to Administer} = \text{Dose Ordered} \times \frac{\text{Prescribed Volume}}{\text{Available Strenght}}$$

This formula provides a consistent method for calculating the correct dose, whether the prescription involves tablets, liquid medications, or injectable solutions.

2. Apply the Formula:

Use the available information to solve for the correct dose. For example:

- If a prescription calls for **250 mg** of a medication and the vial contains **500 mg/2 mL**, the calculation would be:

$$\text{Dose to Administer} = 250\text{ mg} \times \frac{2\text{ mL}}{500\text{ mg}} = 1\text{ mL}$$

This result ensures the client receives the precise amount of medication prescribed.

3. Double-Check the Calculation:

Always cross-verify your calculations, either with a colleague or using a reliable medical calculator. Double-checking is especially critical for high-alert medications, where errors can have severe consequences.

4. Consider Special Populations:

For pediatric clients, weight-based dosing is essential. Begin by converting the client's weight from pounds to kilograms (1 pound = 0.454 kilograms). For example, a child weighing **44 pounds** would be converted to **20 kilograms**. If the prescription is for **5 mg/kg**, the calculation would be:

$$\text{Dose to Administer} = 20\text{ kg} \times 5\,\frac{\text{mg}}{\text{kg}} = 100\text{ mg}$$

This additional step ensures the dose is tailored to the client's specific needs, particularly in populations with narrower therapeutic margins.

5. Context Matters:

In infusion rate calculations, consider factors like the prescribed rate, tubing drop factor, and infusion time. For instance, calculating drops per minute for an IV order of **125 mL/hour** with a drop factor of **15 drops/mL** involves:

$$\text{Drops per Minute} = \frac{125 \text{ mL/hour} \times 15 \text{ gtt/mL}}{60 \text{ min/hour}} = 31.25 \text{ gtt/mL}$$

Rounded to **31 drops/minute**, this ensures the client receives the correct infusion rate.

Error Prevention Strategies

Beyond performing calculations, adhering to robust error prevention measures is essential:

- **Follow the Rights of Medication Administration:**

  Verify the right client, medication, dose, route, time, documentation, and reason every time you prepare and administer medications. These checks form the foundation of safe pharmacological practice.
- **Double-Check High-Risk Situations:**

  Pay special attention to high-alert medications or prescriptions for vulnerable populations, such as pediatric or geriatric clients. Errors in these cases can have amplified consequences.
- **Consult Institutional Protocols:**

  Refer to facility-specific policies, which often include safeguards like independent double-checks for certain medications or weight-based dosing guidelines.

Practice Scenarios for Reinforcement

To solidify understanding, practical examples and exercises are invaluable:

- **Example 1: Pediatric Dosing**

  A child weighing **15 kilograms** is prescribed a medication at **10 mg/kg/day**, divided into two doses. The total daily dose is:

$$\text{Dose per Day} = 15 \text{ kg} \times 10 \text{ mg/kg/day} = 150 \text{ mg}$$

Dividing this into two doses gives **75 mg per dose**, ensuring accurate administration.

- **Example 2: Infusion Rate Calculation**

  For an IV order of **250 mL over 2 hours** using tubing with a drop factor of **20 drops/mL**, calculate the drops per minute:

$$\text{Drops per Minute} = \frac{250 \times 20}{60 \times 2} = \frac{5000}{120} = 41.67 \text{ gtt/mL}$$

  Rounded to **42 drops/minute**, this ensures the client receives the prescribed infusion accurately.

6.2 Educating and Monitoring Clients on Medication Use

Effective client education and diligent monitoring are essential to ensure the safe and effective use of medications. Nurses play a critical role in bridging the gap between medical recommendations and the client's understanding, ensuring adherence to therapeutic regimens and minimizing adverse effects. This section highlights strategies for educating clients on pharmacological management and monitoring their responses to medication, particularly in conditions like Meniere's disease, where treatment adherence is key to improving quality of life.

Effective client education hinges on clear and accessible communication. Nurses should prioritize using simple, client-friendly language to explain the purpose and mechanisms of medications. For instance, when discussing antiemetics for Meniere's disease, a nurse might explain that these medications "reduce the signals in the brain that cause nausea," helping clients feel more capable of managing their symptoms. This approach demystifies the medication and builds client confiidence in the treatment.

Visual aids, such as charts or medication schedules, can further enhance understanding, particularly for clients managing multiple prescriptions. These tools serve as easy-to-follow references, ensuring clients feel equipped to maintain their medication regimen at home. Incorporating relatable analogies also helps simplify complex concepts. For example, diuretics can be described as "helping your body get rid of extra water, making it easier for your heart and blood vessels to work properly."

Providing written handouts or digital resources, such as videos or online guides, ensures that clients can revisit important information at their convenience. This is especially helpful for those who may feel overwhelmed during the initial teaching session.

Educating clients about potential side effects is essential for fostering adherence and preventing complications. Nurses should empower clients to recognize early signs of adverse reactions and take appropriate action. For example:

- **Antiemetics:** Clients should be advised to monitor for excessive sedation or confusion, as these may signal the need for a dosage adjustment.
- **Diuretics:** Encourage clients to watch for dehydration symptoms, such as dry mouth, dizziness, or reduced urine output, and to stay hydrated while following their prescribed regimen.

Encouraging clients to maintain a symptom and medication diary can be an effective strategy for tracking their responses to treatment. By documenting any side effects, patterns, or improvements, clients can provide valuable insights during follow-up visits. This proactive approach not only helps clients feel more involved in their care but also enables nurses to assess treatment efficacy and adjust the plan as needed.

Follow-up visits are critical for assessing adherence, evaluating therapeutic responses, and addressing any challenges the client may be facing. Nurses should emphasize the importance of these visits as opportunities to refine the care plan and ensure it aligns with the client's evolving needs.

Open communication during follow-ups is key. Nurses should create a supportive environment where clients feel comfortable sharing their experiences, including any barriers to adherence or concerns about side effects. For example, a client who reports nausea as a side effect might benefit from tailored advice, such as taking their medication with a light meal or at a different time of day to reduce discomfort.

Regular follow-ups also reinforce the nurse-client relationship, helping clients feel supported and valued in their journey toward better health. This collaborative approach not only improves medication adherence but also enhances overall treatment outcomes by ensuring the care plan remains responsive and client-centered.

6.3 Medication Safety and Documentation

Medication safety is a fundamental aspect of nursing practice, encompassing not only routine drug administration but also the careful management of medications during specialized diagnostic tests, such as the Tensilon test for diagnosing Myasthenia Gravis. This test, which involves administering edrophonium chloride (Tensilon), carries the risk of inducing a cholinergic crisis—a potentially life-threatening condition. Nurses must be prepared to address such emergencies with precise protocols, including the availability of Atropine sulfate as an antidote.

Medication Safety Protocols

Ensuring medication safety during diagnostic tests requires adherence to strict protocols. Before administering Tensilon, nurses must confirm the availability of Atropine sulfate and verify its correct dosage. Atropine acts rapidly to counteract the effects of excessive acetylcholine, which can cause symptoms such as severe bradycardia, respiratory distress, or muscle weakness during a cholinergic crisis. This preparation ensures that life-saving measures can be implemented without delay.

Documentation is another critical component of medication safety. Nurses must record the precise dosage and timing of Tensilon administration, as well as any use of Atropine. Observations of the client's response to the medication should be detailed, including improvements in muscle strength (indicating a positive test result) or any adverse reactions that occur. This meticulous documentation not only supports the continuity of care but also provides a clear record for evaluating the test's outcome and any necessary interventions.

Monitoring and Client Safety

Close monitoring of the client during and after the Tensilon test is essential to ensure safety. Nurses should observe for signs of adverse reactions, such as bradycardia, hypotension, or respiratory distress, which may indicate a cholinergic crisis. Immediate intervention with Atropine is required in such cases, alongside supportive measures like oxygen therapy or airway management if needed.

Educating clients about the Tensilon test is equally important for promoting safety and building trust. Nurses should explain the test's purpose—to evaluate muscle strength in suspected cases of

Myasthenia Gravis—and outline potential risks, such as the possibility of adverse reactions. Reassuring clients about the presence of emergency measures, including the readiness of Atropine and continuous monitoring, helps alleviate anxiety and ensures their informed consent.

In addition to real-time safety measures, proactive communication and preparation are vital. Nurses should collaborate with the healthcare team to ensure that all necessary equipment, such as a cardiac monitor and resuscitation tools, is readily available. This collaborative approach minimizes risks and ensures that the test proceeds smoothly.

6.4 Administration Techniques Across Routes

Medication administration involves a variety of techniques tailored to specific routes, each with unique considerations to ensure efficacy and client safety. This section focuses on the range of administration methods, emphasizing specialized techniques like intrathecal medication delivery, which plays a critical role in managing complex conditions such as metastases, chronic pain, or cerebrospinal infections. By understanding the indications, procedures, and nursing considerations for these routes, nurses can ensure precision and safety in their practice.

6.4.1 Intrathecal Administration Overview

Intrathecal administration is a highly specialized and precise method of delivering medications directly into the cerebrospinal fluid (CSF) via a lumbar puncture or an implanted catheter. By bypassing the blood-brain barrier, this technique ensures that medications act directly on the central nervous system (CNS), making it an invaluable option in managing certain complex medical conditions. Its ability to target the CNS with minimal systemic exposure reduces the likelihood of widespread side effects, enhancing both safety and efficacy.

This route is particularly beneficial in situations where traditional methods of drug delivery are inadequate. Common scenarios include:

- **Chronic Pain Management:** Intrathecal analgesics are used for clients with severe, refractory pain that cannot be effectively managed through oral or systemic opioid therapy. This targeted delivery provides potent relief while minimizing the systemic side effects associated with higher doses of opioids.
- **CNS Infections:** Conditions like meningitis often require high local concentrations of antibiotics to combat the infection effectively. Intrathecal administration ensures the antibiotics reach the infected area directly, overcoming limitations posed by the blood-brain barrier.
- **Chemotherapy for CNS Metastases:** When cancer metastasizes to the brain or spinal cord, systemic chemotherapy may struggle to reach therapeutic levels in the CNS. Intrathecal delivery allows for direct treatment of these metastases, improving outcomes in clients with advanced cancer.

In addition to these applications, intrathecal administration is also used for delivering certain anesthetics during surgeries or labor, offering rapid and localized pain relief.

The precision of intrathecal administration makes it a powerful tool, but it also requires careful handling and specialized training. This route demands meticulous attention to sterile technique, as any contamination can lead to serious complications, including meningitis or abscess formation. Nurses play a crucial role in preparing for and monitoring these procedures, ensuring that both the medication and the delivery method align with the client's specific needs.

For example, in a client with metastatic cancer, the use of intrathecal chemotherapy not only reduces tumor growth but also minimizes the systemic toxicity that would occur if the same drugs were administered intravenously. Similarly, a client with bacterial meningitis receiving intrathecal antibiotics may experience quicker resolution of symptoms due to the localized and effective drug concentration in the CSF.

6.4.2 Nursing Considerations for Intrathecal Administration

The complexity and precision required for intrathecal administration demand exceptional attention to detail and a thorough understanding of potential risks. One of the most critical aspects of this procedure is maintaining a sterile technique. Since intrathecal administration directly involves the central nervous system (CNS), any lapse in sterility can result in severe complications, such as meningitis or abscess formation. Nurses must rigorously ensure that all equipment, including needles, catheters, and medication vials, is sterile, and that the procedure environment is free from contamination. Proper client positioning—typically in a lateral decubitus or sitting position—is essential to facilitate safe access to the cerebrospinal fluid (CSF) and ensure client comfort during the procedure.

Close monitoring of clients after intrathecal administration is equally critical, as adverse effects can arise quickly. Key areas for observation include:

- **Infection:** Nurses should remain vigilant for signs such as fever, redness, swelling at the injection site, or general malaise, which may indicate an infection. Early detection is crucial to prevent further complications.
- **Neurologic Changes:** Adverse effects on the CNS, such as altered mental status, severe headaches, sensory deficits, or weakness, require immediate attention. These changes may signal complications like increased intracranial pressure or nerve damage.
- **CSF Leakage:** Post-procedure headaches, especially those exacerbated by standing and alleviated by lying down, can indicate a CSF leak at the puncture site. Nurses should monitor for this and provide appropriate interventions, such as hydration or advising the client to remain in a reclined position.

Client education plays a significant role in promoting safety and reducing anxiety. Clear communication about the procedure and its potential effects helps clients feel informed and prepared. For example, nurses can explain:

- **What to Expect During the Procedure:** Reassure clients that while they may feel brief discomfort or pressure during the lumbar puncture, the procedure is generally well-tolerated and temporary.
- **Post-Procedure Care:** Educate clients about potential side effects, such as mild headaches or localized soreness, and provide guidance on managing these symptoms. For example, encourage hydration to reduce the likelihood of headaches and explain when to report symptoms like prolonged pain or fever.
- **When to Seek Medical Attention:** Provide clear instructions on recognizing and reporting serious complications, such as persistent headaches, signs of infection, or unusual neurologic symptoms.

6.4.3 Comparisons with Other Routes

Intrathecal administration stands apart from other medication delivery routes such as intravenous (IV), rectal, or intramuscular (IM) in its ability to deliver drugs directly to the central nervous system (CNS) with unparalleled precision. While IV administration is a mainstay for systemic delivery due to its rapid absorption and distribution throughout the body, it cannot bypass the blood-brain barrier. Intrathecal administration, by contrast, introduces medications directly into the cerebrospinal fluid (CSF), allowing for higher concentrations of the drug at the target site and minimizing systemic side effects.

Rectal and intramuscular routes, although less invasive, also fall short in terms of precision and efficacy for CNS-targeted therapies. Rectal administration is typically reserved for clients who cannot take medications orally, but its absorption is inconsistent and influenced by factors like rectal blood flow and motility. IM injections provide relatively steady absorption but are not suitable for conditions requiring direct CNS intervention.

The advantages of intrathecal administration are best understood through real-world scenarios:

- **Targeted Pain Management in Metastatic Cancer:** Clients with metastatic cancer often suffer from debilitating spinal pain that systemic opioids may not adequately relieve. Intrathecal analgesics, such as morphine, can deliver potent pain relief directly to the CNS, reducing the risk of sedation and other systemic side effects associated with high-dose opioids.
- **Treating Bacterial Meningitis:** In cases of bacterial meningitis, where rapid and effective antibiotic delivery is critical, intrathecal administration allows for high concentrations of the medication directly in the CSF, ensuring swift action against the infection and improving client outcomes.

While intrathecal administration offers distinct benefits, it also carries inherent risks, such as infection or neurologic complications, requiring meticulous technique and monitoring. By understanding how it compares to other routes, nurses can make informed decisions about when this specialized method is appropriate and ensure its safe and effective implementation. This knowledge underscores the importance of tailoring medication delivery to the specific needs and conditions of each client, optimizing both efficacy and safety.

6.5 Intravenous and Blood Product Administration

Intravenous (IV) therapy is a cornerstone of modern medical care, used for fluid replacement, medication delivery, and blood product transfusions. Proper administration techniques and vigilant monitoring are critical to ensuring client safety and achieving therapeutic outcomes. This section provides an in-depth exploration of safe IV practices, the management of complications, and emergency preparedness, focusing on both routine care and critical situations like anaphylaxis.

6.5.1 General Considerations for Intravenous and Blood Product Administration

Intravenous (IV) therapy, whether for delivering fluids, medications, or blood products, requires precision, vigilance, and strict adherence to safety protocols. Because IV administration involves direct access to the bloodstream, the margin for error is minimal, making attention to detail critical. Nurses play a pivotal role in ensuring that every step, from preparation to monitoring, is conducted correctly to maximize therapeutic benefits while minimizing risks.

Proper catheter placement is the cornerstone of effective IV therapy. Before initiating the infusion, nurses must confirm that the IV site is patent and free of complications such as infiltration or phlebitis. Maintaining aseptic technique is essential throughout the process to prevent infections, which can have severe consequences, especially for immunocompromised clients. Frequent assessment of the IV site is also necessary to identify early signs of complications like redness, swelling, or pain.

When administering blood products, additional safety measures must be observed. The compatibility of the blood product with the client's blood type must be verified meticulously to prevent hemolytic reactions. Double-checking orders, performing baseline vital sign assessments, and closely monitoring the client during the transfusion are vital to detect early signs of adverse reactions. For example, fever, chills, or flank pain may indicate a transfusion reaction, which requires immediate intervention to prevent escalation.

Another critical aspect is the documentation of all procedures. Accurate and comprehensive records not only provide a clear history of the client's care but also ensure accountability and continuity of care. Every step, from verifying the client's identity to monitoring their response, should be recorded in detail.

Key considerations for IV and blood product administration include:

- **Verifying orders, identity, and compatibility:** Confirm that the physician's orders match the client's condition and that the correct fluid or product is being administered. This step is especially important for high-risk infusions, such as blood products or chemotherapy agents.
- **Monitoring infusion rates:** Infusion rates should be carefully calibrated, particularly for vulnerable populations like pediatric or elderly clients who may be at higher risk for fluid overload. Using infusion pumps or controllers helps ensure precision in delivery.
- **Observing for complications:** Regularly assess the client for signs of infiltration (e.g., swelling, coolness, or pain at the site) or phlebitis (e.g., warmth, redness, or a palpable cord). Early detection allows for timely intervention, preventing further complications.
- **Education and communication:** Educate clients about the procedure, including what they can expect and what symptoms to report. Clear communication reduces anxiety and encourages clients to participate in their care.

In blood product administration, ensuring compatibility extends beyond simply matching blood types. Nurses must also check the expiration date and storage conditions of the blood product and confirm the presence of informed consent before beginning the transfusion. Close observation during the initial 15 minutes of the transfusion is critical, as most adverse reactions occur during this time.

6.5.2 Recognizing and Responding to Anaphylaxis

Anaphylaxis represents one of the most critical emergencies that can arise during IV medication administration or blood product transfusion. This severe allergic reaction requires immediate recognition and intervention to prevent life-threatening consequences. Nurses are often the first to detect the early signs, which include a combination of systemic symptoms such as hypotension, tachycardia, respiratory distress, and visible skin manifestations like hives, flushing, or angioedema (swelling of the face, lips, or tongue).

In many cases, respiratory symptoms such as wheezing or stridor indicate airway compromise, while hypotension and rapid pulse suggest cardiovascular collapse. The rapid onset and progression of anaphylaxis underscore the importance of swift and decisive action. Early recognition is the cornerstone of effective management, as delays in intervention can lead to fatal outcomes.

The primary nursing response to suspected anaphylaxis is to stop the IV flow immediately to halt further exposure to the triggering allergen. Keeping the IV line patent by running normal saline is essential, as it provides a direct route for administering emergency medications. Nurses should notify the healthcare provider without delay while simultaneously initiating emergency protocols.

Administering epinephrine is the first-line treatment for anaphylaxis. Epinephrine works by reversing the life-threatening effects of the allergic reaction, including airway constriction, hypotension, and swelling. Nurses must administer this medication promptly, following established dosing guidelines, and closely monitor the client for any response. Oxygen therapy may be necessary to address hypoxia, and antihistamines or corticosteroids may be administered as prescribed to address residual symptoms and prevent recurrence.

Additional steps for managing anaphylaxis include:

- **Maintaining airway patency:** Continuously assess the client's breathing, watching for signs of obstruction. Be prepared to use suction devices or assist with intubation if needed.
- **Monitoring vital signs:** Regularly check blood pressure, heart rate, oxygen saturation, and respiratory rate to evaluate the effectiveness of interventions and detect any further deterioration.
- **Preparing for complications:** Have emergency equipment, such as a bag-valve mask, defibrillator, and advanced airway supplies, readily available in case of cardiopulmonary arrest.
- **Providing emotional support:** Reassure the client and their family throughout the process, explaining each step being taken to manage the reaction.

Education and preparedness are key in minimizing the risks associated with anaphylaxis. Nurses should ensure that emergency supplies, such as epinephrine, oxygen, and suction equipment, are readily accessible in areas where IV medications or blood transfusions are administered. Additionally, reviewing the client's allergy history before starting any infusion can help identify potential risks and guide preemptive safety measures.

6.5.3 Emergency Preparedness

Emergency preparedness is a vital component of safe and effective IV therapy, ensuring that nurses can respond promptly and effectively to life-threatening complications. IV therapy, particularly when administering high-risk medications or performing blood transfusions, carries inherent risks such as anaphylaxis, air embolisms, or severe transfusion reactions. Being ready to manage these emergencies not only safeguards client safety but also reinforces trust in the healthcare team.

Having immediate access to emergency equipment and medications is non-negotiable. Supplies such as epinephrine, antihistamines, corticosteroids, and oxygen should always be within reach, especially when administering medications with a high potential for adverse reactions. For example, during blood transfusions, keeping epinephrine readily available ensures a rapid response to anaphylactic reactions. Oxygen tanks, suction devices, and intravenous fluids for resuscitation should also be accessible and checked regularly to confirm their functionality.

Familiarity with institutional protocols is equally critical. Nurses must be well-versed in the steps for managing IV-related emergencies, such as stopping the infusion immediately, maintaining a patent IV line for administering emergency medications, and escalating care by notifying the healthcare provider or rapid response team. Regular training sessions and simulations can help ensure that nurses are confident in implementing these protocols under pressure.

Key strategies for enhancing emergency preparedness include:

- **Proactive Planning:** Before initiating high-risk IV therapy, nurses should review the client's medical history for potential allergies, previous transfusion reactions, or sensitivities to specific medications. This information allows for tailored precautions, such as premedication with antihistamines or closer monitoring during the infusion.
- **Clear Communication:** Educating clients about what to expect during IV therapy can aid in early identification of complications. For instance, advising clients to report symptoms like itching, difficulty breathing, or a metallic taste in their mouth can expedite intervention during an adverse reaction.
- **Team Collaboration:** Emergency preparedness is a team effort. All staff involved in IV therapy should be educated on recognizing early signs of complications, such as hypotension, tachycardia, or cyanosis, and know how to respond efficiently. Coordinated drills and clear role assignments during emergencies ensure that every team member contributes effectively to resolving the situation.

Documentation is another critical aspect of emergency preparedness. Nurses must thoroughly record all observations, interventions, and client responses during and after an emergency. This documentation not only supports continuity of care but also provides valuable insights for quality improvement and legal accountability. For example, noting the exact time a transfusion reaction began, the interventions performed, and the client's subsequent condition helps refine protocols and ensures accurate reporting to the interdisciplinary team.

6.6 Pain Management and Specialized Devices

Effective pain management is a cornerstone of nursing care, particularly for clients with chronic pain or those using specialized devices like patient-controlled analgesia (PCA) pumps. This section explores the concept of drug tolerance, strategies for managing chronic pain, and approaches to educating clients and families. By understanding these elements, nurses can ensure that pain is managed effectively while minimizing risks and fostering trust in the care process.

6.6.1 Understanding Drug Tolerance

Drug tolerance is a physiological phenomenon in which the body becomes less responsive to a medication over time, requiring higher doses to achieve the same therapeutic effect. This adaptation is especially common in clients with chronic pain who rely on long-term analgesic therapy. Understanding the distinction between drug tolerance and drug addiction is critical to preventing unnecessary stigma and ensuring clients receive the compassionate care they need. Tolerance is a natural, expected response to prolonged medication use, whereas addiction involves compulsive behavior, psychological dependence, and misuse, which are separate from tolerance.

For instance, a client taking opioids for chronic back pain may notice that their initial dose no longer provides adequate relief after several months. This does not indicate misuse or addiction but reflects the body's physiological adjustment to the medication. Such situations highlight the importance of educating clients and caregivers about drug tolerance to alleviate fears or misconceptions about the need for dosage adjustments.

Nurses play a pivotal role in addressing these changes with empathy and professionalism. Collaborative care planning ensures that clients continue to receive effective pain relief while maintaining trust in the healthcare team. Regular assessments of pain levels and medication efficacy allow for timely adjustments to the treatment plan, whether through increasing dosages, rotating to a different medication, or integrating nonpharmacological pain management strategies.

It is equally important to validate clients' experiences with chronic pain and reassure them that requiring higher doses is not a sign of failure or a moral issue but rather a normal response to long-term therapy. This understanding fosters a supportive environment where clients feel heard and respected, reducing the anxiety often associated with medication adjustments. By addressing drug tolerance with expertise and compassion, nurses can help clients navigate their pain management journey with confidence and dignity.

6.6.2 Managing Pain in Clients with Drug Tolerance

Managing chronic pain in clients with drug tolerance requires a comprehensive and individualized approach to ensure effective relief while minimizing potential risks. One widely used strategy is opioid rotation, where the client transitions to a different opioid medication to leverage differences in drug metabolism and receptor binding. This method helps "reset" tolerance levels, allowing for improved pain control without significantly increasing the dosage of any single medication. For example, a client who has developed tolerance to morphine may experience better relief by switching to hydromorphone, as their body may respond differently to the new drug.

Integrating nonpharmacological methods into the pain management plan is equally critical. Techniques such as physical therapy, guided relaxation, mindfulness practices, and cognitive-behavioral therapy (CBT) provide holistic support, addressing both the physical and emotional dimensions of chronic pain. For instance, physical therapy can improve mobility and reduce muscle tension, while mindfulness exercises help clients focus on managing their pain with greater resilience. CBT, in particular, is effective in reshaping negative thought patterns associated with chronic pain, fostering a sense of control and well-being.

Regular and open communication between nurses and clients is a cornerstone of successful pain management in cases of drug tolerance. Nurses should consistently evaluate pain levels using standardized scales and seek client feedback about medication efficacy and side effects. Encouraging clients to share their experiences openly not only builds trust but also ensures timely adjustments to their care plan. For example, if a client reports diminished relief from their current medication, this dialogue allows the nurse to advocate for changes, such as adjusting the dose, switching medications, or incorporating new therapeutic approaches.

In addition, educating clients about the concept of drug tolerance and the available strategies to address it helps alleviate fears of dependence or addiction. Reassuring clients that tolerance is a normal physiological response and explaining the rationale for adjustments in their treatment plan can reduce anxiety and promote adherence. By adopting a proactive, empathetic, and collaborative approach, nurses can empower clients to manage their chronic pain effectively and improve their quality of life.

6.6.3 Client Education and Alleviating Concerns

Educating clients and their families about drug tolerance and chronic pain management is essential to fostering trust, ensuring adherence, and alleviating unnecessary concerns. Misconceptions about drug tolerance often lead to fears of addiction, making it crucial for nurses to provide clear, empathetic explanations. Many clients and families may not understand the difference between tolerance and addiction, so addressing this distinction is a key part of the education process.

For instance, nurses can explain drug tolerance in simple terms: "When you take a medication for a long time, your body can get used to it. That's why we might need to adjust the dose or try a different medication. This is not addiction—it's a natural response of the body." Reassuring clients about adjustments to their pain management plan is equally important: "Sometimes, managing chronic pain means making small changes to your treatment. These adjustments help us keep your pain under control in the safest and most effective way."

Emphasizing the importance of adherence to prescribed medications helps clients understand that following their plan reduces risks and enhances outcomes. Clients should be reassured that their healthcare team monitors them closely to address any changes in their condition or response to treatment. Written materials, diagrams, or visual aids that detail drug tolerance and chronic pain management strategies can reinforce verbal education, providing a reference for clients and families to revisit as needed.

Encouraging clients to actively engage in their care by maintaining a pain diary is another valuable strategy. This diary can include details about pain levels, medication timing, and any side effects experienced. Such documentation not only empowers clients by increasing their awareness of patterns in their pain but also provides the healthcare team with critical insights during follow-up visits. These insights allow for a more tailored approach to pain management, ensuring that clients feel heard and supported.

Chapter 7
Reduction of risk potential

This chapter focuses on strategies to minimize risks and prevent complications in client care. Nurses play a crucial role in identifying potential hazards, implementing safety measures, and ensuring effective monitoring during diagnostic procedures and treatments. By mastering these skills, nurses can reduce the likelihood of adverse outcomes and provide high-quality, client-centered care.

Key topics include the proper monitoring of vital signs, understanding diagnostic test results, maintaining invasive devices, and educating clients about procedures and treatments. These foundational competencies enable nurses to anticipate and address potential risks, ensuring the best possible outcomes in diverse clinical scenarios.

7.1 Monitoring and Collecting Client Data

Monitoring and collecting client data are fundamental nursing responsibilities that ensure early detection of potential health issues and support accurate diagnoses. This section covers essential techniques for obtaining vital signs, performing electrocardiograms (EKG/ECG), and collecting diagnostic specimens. Nurses must approach these tasks with precision and attention to detail, as errors in data collection or interpretation can lead to missed or delayed interventions.

7.1.1 Monitoring Vital Signs

Vital signs offer a critical snapshot of a client's overall health, serving as early indicators of potential changes in their condition. Accurate measurement and interpretation of temperature, pulse, respiration, blood pressure, and oxygen saturation are essential for timely interventions and effective care. Nurses must adhere to standardized techniques to ensure reliability and minimize errors in data collection.

For blood pressure, using the correct cuff size is vital, as an improperly sized cuff can lead to inaccurate readings. A cuff that is too small may result in falsely elevated readings, while one that is too large can underestimate true blood pressure values. When measuring respirations, careful observation of rate, depth, and effort is necessary. Signs of respiratory distress, such as shallow breathing, use of accessory muscles, or audible wheezing, should prompt immediate assessment and intervention.

Monitoring oxygen saturation with a pulse oximeter requires careful attention to sensor placement. Poor placement or interference, such as cold extremities or nail polish, can cause false readings. It is equally important to recheck values that fall outside normal ranges to confirm accuracy before initiating interventions. For example, a low oxygen saturation reading (below 92%) may indicate hypoxemia, necessitating supplemental oxygen or further evaluation to address underlying causes.

Understanding the normal ranges for vital signs and recognizing deviations are crucial to effective nursing practice. A pulse rate above 100 beats per minute (tachycardia) might signal conditions like fever, dehydration, or pain, while bradycardia (a rate below 60 beats per minute) could indicate heart block or effects of certain medications. Similarly, a temperature above 100.4°F (38°C) may signify infection, while hypothermia (below 96.8°F or 36°C) could point to systemic shock or exposure.

Accurate and timely documentation plays a pivotal role in monitoring vital signs. Recording each value immediately after measurement ensures that the data is available for comparison over time. Trends, such as a gradual increase in blood pressure or persistent low oxygen saturation, can provide critical insights into a client's condition. Nurses should note any interventions taken and their outcomes, such as the administration of antipyretics for fever or oxygen therapy for hypoxemia.

Additionally, communicating findings effectively with the healthcare team is vital. For example, if a client exhibits tachycardia with accompanying symptoms such as dizziness or shortness of breath, it is crucial to escalate these findings promptly. This proactive approach ensures that potential complications are addressed before they escalate into emergencies.

7.1.2 Performing and Interpreting EKGs

Electrocardiograms (EKGs/ECGs) are vital tools for evaluating cardiac function and detecting abnormalities such as arrhythmias, ischemia, or myocardial infarction. Nurses are instrumental in both performing the procedure accurately and recognizing significant findings that may require urgent intervention.

Proper preparation and electrode placement are fundamental to obtaining a clear and reliable EKG reading. The skin must be cleaned and dried thoroughly to reduce interference from oils or moisture, which can create artifacts on the tracing. Securely attaching the electrodes is equally important to prevent signal disruptions. For a standard 12-lead EKG, nurses must adhere to precise lead placement protocols:

- Place limb leads on the wrists and ankles or their proximal equivalents if needed.
- Position chest leads (V1-V6) at specific intercostal spaces and along the midline of the chest to capture detailed electrical activity of the heart.

Ensuring correct placement not only enhances the quality of the EKG but also prevents false readings that could lead to misinterpretation.

Once the EKG is performed, nurses should promptly review the tracing for basic abnormalities. While a full diagnostic interpretation is typically the responsibility of the physician, nurses must be adept at identifying critical changes, including:

- **Irregular rhythms:** Patterns such as atrial fibrillation, ventricular tachycardia, or asystole are red flags requiring immediate notification of the healthcare provider.
- **ST segment changes:** Elevation may signal acute myocardial infarction, while depression could indicate ischemia. Both findings warrant urgent intervention.
- **Prolonged intervals:** A prolonged QT interval increases the risk of life-threatening arrhythmias like torsades de pointes. Similarly, a lengthened PR interval could signify first-degree heart block.

To ensure client safety, nurses should act swiftly if abnormalities are detected. For example, in cases of suspected myocardial infarction, the nurse should immediately inform the provider and prepare for interventions such as administering oxygen, obtaining additional diagnostic labs (e.g., cardiac enzymes), or initiating protocols for chest pain management.

It is also essential to document the EKG procedure accurately, including the time, reason for the test, and any notable findings observed. This ensures continuity of care and provides a clear record for the healthcare team.

Client education is another important aspect of the EKG process. Nurses should explain the procedure in simple terms, reassuring clients that it is painless and typically quick. For instance, clients undergoing their first EKG may benefit from knowing that the test helps "check the heart's electrical signals to ensure everything is working as it should." Clear communication can reduce anxiety and improve cooperation during the procedure.

7.1.3 Collecting Specimens for Diagnostic Tests

Specimen collection is a fundamental aspect of nursing care, essential for accurate diagnostic results and effective treatment planning. The process requires meticulous attention to detail, as proper technique, sterility, and adherence to protocols are critical to preserving specimen integrity and ensuring reliable test outcomes. Nurses play a pivotal role in collecting various types of specimens, including blood, urine, stool, and sputum, while also addressing client concerns to foster cooperation.

Blood Specimens: Performing venipuncture demands a thorough understanding of aseptic techniques to minimize the risk of infection. Selecting the correct collection tubes, based on the specific tests ordered, is equally important to ensure accurate results. Nurses should label the tubes immediately and clearly, avoiding any risk of misidentification. If multiple tests are ordered, the sequence of tube collection should follow established guidelines to prevent contamination between additives.

Urine Specimens: For midstream clean-catch samples, nurses must provide clients with clear instructions to ensure the collection is free from contamination. In situations requiring sterile samples, catheterization techniques may be necessary. Maintaining sterility throughout the process and ensuring the client's comfort are priorities. Additionally, nurses should explain the need for prompt sample delivery to the lab to prevent degradation.

Stool Specimens: Clients collecting stool samples must be educated on avoiding contamination from toilet water, tissue, or other materials. Providing a clean collection container and clear verbal or written instructions ensures the sample is suitable for analysis. Nurses should also confirm if any dietary restrictions or medications need to be avoided prior to collection, depending on the test.

Sputum Specimens: Sputum collection is most effective in the morning when secretions are concentrated. Clients should be instructed to take deep breaths and cough forcefully to produce samples from the lower respiratory tract, rather than saliva. Nurses can assist by demonstrating the technique and ensuring the collection cup remains sterile throughout the process.

Handling and Education

After collecting the specimens, careful labeling, storage, and timely transportation to the laboratory are crucial to maintaining their viability. Nurses must double-check labels to ensure accuracy, including client name, date, time, and test type. Some specimens may require refrigeration or specific handling to prevent degradation, which should be communicated to the laboratory staff.

Client education is an integral part of specimen collection. Explaining the purpose of the test helps clients understand its importance and reduces anxiety. For example, a nurse might say, "This blood test will help us check your sugar levels to ensure your medication is working effectively." Addressing discomfort or concerns, such as fear of needles or embarrassment about stool or sputum collection, further supports client cooperation and trust.

7.2 Managing Diagnostic and Laboratory Procedures

Managing diagnostic and laboratory procedures is a vital responsibility for nurses, as it ensures accurate results and timely interventions. From interpreting laboratory test outcomes to maintaining critical devices such as central venous catheters (CVCs), nurses play a pivotal role in bridging diagnostic insights with effective care. This section will explore strategies for monitoring test results, maintaining essential medical devices, and performing techniques such as venipuncture and glucose monitoring with precision and adherence to safety standards.

7.2.1 Monitoring and Documenting Diagnostic and Laboratory Test Results

Properly monitoring and documenting diagnostic and laboratory test results is a cornerstone of effective nursing practice. This process is essential for tracking a client's condition, detecting subtle changes, and guiding timely clinical decisions. Nurses must adopt a systematic approach to reviewing test outcomes, identifying abnormalities, and promptly communicating significant findings to the healthcare team to ensure comprehensive and coordinated care.

For instance, reviewing a client's complete blood count (CBC) might reveal elevated white blood cell counts, often signaling an infection or inflammatory response, or decreased hemoglobin levels, which could indicate anemia or blood loss. Similarly, abnormalities in kidney function markers, such as a steady rise in creatinine or blood urea nitrogen (BUN) levels, may point to declining renal function and necessitate immediate intervention. Recognizing these patterns enables nurses to act decisively, ensuring that the client receives appropriate care without delay.

Accurate documentation is equally crucial, as it provides a clear and reliable record for the entire healthcare team. Nurses should:

- Record test results meticulously, including the client's name, date, and time of testing, to prevent errors or misinterpretation.
- Highlight trends or deviations over time, such as a progressive increase in blood glucose levels, which may indicate poorly managed diabetes.
- Detail any interventions undertaken in response to abnormal results, such as notifying the physician, adjusting treatment plans, or monitoring the client for further changes.

Nurses should also be prepared to explain test results to clients and families, offering clear, jargon-free explanations to help them understand the implications of the findings. For example, a nurse might reassure a client with mild electrolyte imbalances by explaining how small dietary adjustments or medications can restore balance.

7.2.2 Central Venous Catheter (CVC) Care

Central venous catheters (CVCs) are vital for clients requiring long-term therapies, such as intravenous medications, total parenteral nutrition (TPN), or fluid administration. While highly effective, their use demands rigorous care and monitoring to minimize risks, particularly catheter-related bloodstream infections (CRBSIs), which can have serious consequences. Nurses play a critical role in ensuring the safe and effective use of CVCs through meticulous care, troubleshooting, and client education.

Infection Prevention

Preventing infection is a top priority in CVC care. Adherence to sterile technique during dressing changes, including using sterile gloves, masks, and disinfectants like chlorhexidine, is essential. Regular flushing of the catheter with saline or heparin, as prescribed, helps maintain patency and reduces the risk of blockages. Nurses should frequently inspect the insertion site for signs of infection, such as redness, swelling, tenderness, or drainage, and document findings accurately. Prompt recognition and intervention are critical to stopping infections before they progress.

Troubleshooting Complications

Nurses must be vigilant in identifying and resolving potential complications with CVCs. For instance:

- **Clots or Obstructions:** Difficulty flushing the catheter or sluggish blood return may indicate a blockage, requiring protocols such as administering a thrombolytic agent or repositioning the catheter.
- **Air Embolism:** While rare, air entering the catheter can be life-threatening. Nurses should ensure the catheter is clamped or capped properly during any disconnections.
- **Mechanical Issues:** Cracked or damaged lines should be reported immediately to prevent leakage or compromised functionality.

Client and Caregiver Education

Educating clients and their caregivers about proper CVC care enhances safety and empowers them to participate in their treatment. Key points include:

- Recognizing signs of infection, such as fever, chills, or increased discomfort around the insertion site.
- Understanding the importance of keeping the catheter site clean and dry and reporting any unusual occurrences promptly.
- Following guidelines for handling the catheter at home, including proper flushing techniques and precautions during daily activities to prevent accidental dislodgement.

7.2.3 Performing Venipuncture and Glucose Monitoring

Venipuncture and glucose monitoring are integral components of nursing practice, requiring a blend of technical precision and client-centered care. These procedures not only provide critical diagnostic information but also offer opportunities to educate clients and build trust.

Venipuncture Techniques

Performing venipuncture involves skillfully obtaining blood samples while prioritizing client comfort and safety. Nurses must:

- **Vein Selection:** Assess the client's veins for size, location, and accessibility. Common sites include the antecubital fossa or dorsal hand veins, chosen based on the purpose of the test and the client's condition.
- **Aseptic Technique:** Maintain sterility throughout the procedure to prevent contamination or infection. This includes proper hand hygiene, using sterile equipment, and cleaning the puncture site with an appropriate antiseptic.
- **Minimizing Discomfort:** Engage clients in relaxation techniques, such as deep breathing or conversation, to reduce anxiety and discomfort. For pediatric or anxious clients, distraction

tools or numbing agents may also be used. For example, when conducting a glucose tolerance test, precise timing and accurate labeling of each sample are essential to ensure reliable results and support effective clinical decision-making.

Glucose Monitoring

Glucose monitoring plays a vital role in managing diabetes and other metabolic conditions. Nurses must ensure accuracy and consistency in this process:

- **Equipment Calibration:** Regularly calibrate glucometers according to manufacturer guidelines to maintain precise readings. Faulty equipment can lead to mismanagement of blood glucose levels.
- **Sample Collection:** Use proper technique when obtaining a capillary blood sample, typically from the lateral side of the fingertip. Ensure the client's hands are clean and warm to improve blood flow and sample quality.
- **Client Education:** Teach clients to monitor their blood glucose levels at home effectively. This includes demonstrating proper strip handling, device maintenance, and disposal of sharps. Education should also cover recognizing symptoms of hypo- or hyperglycemia, such as dizziness, confusion, or excessive thirst, and knowing when to seek medical help.

7.3 Surgical and Invasive Procedure Support

Supporting clients through surgical and invasive procedures requires a comprehensive approach that prioritizes safety, education, and comfort. Nurses play a pivotal role in preparing clients for procedures, providing assistance during interventions, and ensuring effective recovery post-procedure. These responsibilities involve maintaining sterility, reinforcing client education, and implementing strategies to prevent complications.

7.3.1 Preparing Clients for Procedures

Preparation is a crucial aspect of ensuring a successful procedure, as it not only addresses the client's physical requirements but also their emotional well-being. Nurses are central to this process, helping clients feel informed, prepared, and reassured.

Reinforce Education

Providing clear, concise instructions is essential for reducing uncertainty and fostering cooperation. Nurses should use simple, client-friendly language to explain the procedure's purpose and steps. For example, when discussing the insertion of a nasogastric tube, describe how the tube will relieve nausea or abdominal discomfort by removing excess stomach contents. Visual aids or handouts can further enhance understanding, especially for clients who may feel overwhelmed by verbal explanations alone. This step empowers clients, making them active participants in their care.

Address Concerns

Acknowledging and addressing client anxieties is vital for building trust and reducing fear. For instance, clients may express nervousness about discomfort during urinary catheter insertion. Nurses should listen empathetically and offer reassurance, emphasizing that any pain or discomfort will be minimized through careful technique and supportive measures. Encouraging clients to share their concerns not only eases their emotional burden but also helps nurses tailor care to individual needs, creating a more personalized and comforting experience.

Ensure Readiness

Physical preparation is just as important as emotional preparation. Nurses must verify that all necessary pre-procedure steps have been completed. This includes ensuring the client has fasted for the required duration, received any prescribed pre-medications, and avoided contraindicated activities, such as taking anticoagulants before certain surgeries. It's also essential to confirm that informed consent forms are signed and that diagnostics, like lab results or imaging, are available to guide the procedure. Nurses play a key role in coordinating these elements, acting as a final safeguard against errors or omissions.

7.3.2 Inserting, Maintaining, and Removing Devices

The insertion, maintenance, and removal of medical devices such as urinary catheters, nasogastric (NG) tubes, and peripheral IVs are fundamental nursing responsibilities that require precision, vigilance, and client-centered care. Proper management of these devices not only ensures therapeutic efficacy but also minimizes the risk of complications and enhances client comfort.

Urinary Catheters

When inserting urinary catheters, aseptic technique is essential to prevent catheter-associated urinary tract infections (CAUTIs). Nurses should ensure that all equipment is sterile and handle the catheter with care during insertion. Once the catheter is in place, monitoring its function is critical. Regularly check for proper drainage and assess for complications, such as blockages, discomfort, or leakage. When removing the catheter, explain the process to the client to reduce anxiety and discomfort. Encourage adequate fluid intake to help the client resume normal bladder function, and monitor for signs of urinary retention or infection post-removal.

Nasogastric Tubes

NG tubes are frequently used for feeding, medication administration, or stomach decompression. Ensuring correct placement is paramount to prevent complications such as aspiration. Nurses should confirm tube placement using pH testing of gastric aspirate or imaging when required. Regular assessments should include checking for tube patency and monitoring for client discomfort, such as nasal irritation or a sore throat. Providing comfort measures, such as applying a water-soluble lubricant around the nostrils or offering lozenges, can alleviate discomfort. Documentation of all interventions, including placement verification and care provided, is critical for continuity of care.

Peripheral IVs

Peripheral IVs are a common method for delivering fluids, medications, or nutrients directly into the bloodstream. Nurses must monitor the insertion site for any signs of complications, such as redness, swelling, pain, or leakage, which could indicate infiltration, phlebitis, or infection. Maintaining IV flow rates as prescribed is crucial for therapeutic effectiveness and client safety. Additionally, nurses should educate clients on how to avoid dislodging the IV, such as minimizing movement near the site. During removal, ensure a gentle technique to minimize discomfort and inspect the site for any signs of irritation or bleeding.

7.3.3 Preventing Injury and Complications

Ensuring client safety during and after procedures is a critical nursing responsibility that requires a proactive approach and meticulous attention to detail. Implementing preventive measures and monitoring for complications are essential to protect clients from harm and promote smooth recovery.

Preventing Injuries

Nurses play a vital role in minimizing the risk of injury by using proper techniques and providing physical support during client movement. For instance, after procedures involving sedation or anesthesia, clients may experience dizziness or impaired motor coordination. Supporting them during transfers or repositioning helps prevent falls or strain. Proper body mechanics, such as bending at the knees and keeping the back straight, are equally important for nurses to avoid personal injury while assisting clients. Additionally, ensuring that the client's environment is free from hazards, such as loose wires or clutter, further reduces the risk of accidents.

Monitoring for Complications

Vigilant observation for early signs of complications can make a significant difference in client outcomes. After invasive procedures, nurses should closely monitor for indicators such as excessive bleeding, infection, or changes in vital signs. For example:

- **Bleeding:** Check surgical or catheter insertion sites for excessive drainage or hematoma formation.
- **Infection:** Look for redness, warmth, swelling, or discharge around wounds or insertion sites, and monitor for systemic signs like fever.
- **Pneumothorax or air embolism:** After central line insertion, assess for symptoms such as sudden shortness of breath, chest pain, or a drop in oxygen saturation. Promptly reporting and addressing these signs ensures timely interventions that prevent the escalation of complications.

Promoting Recovery

Encouraging clients to participate in activities that support recovery is equally important. Early ambulation, when medically appropriate, is a key strategy to prevent complications such as deep vein thrombosis (DVT) and improve circulation. Nurses should assist clients in safely getting out of bed and provide clear instructions on how to move comfortably after surgery. Breathing exercises, such as incentive spirometry or deep-breathing techniques, help expand the lungs and reduce the risk of atelectasis, particularly after abdominal or thoracic procedures. These small but impactful actions contribute to faster healing and improved outcomes.

7.4 Monitoring and Responding to Client Conditions

Monitoring and responding to client conditions is a cornerstone of safe and effective nursing care. Continuous observation allows nurses to identify subtle changes in a client's status, enabling timely interventions that prevent complications and support recovery. This section emphasizes critical areas of monitoring, including oxygen saturation, nasogastric tube management, and documenting outcomes to guide corrective actions when necessary.

7.4.1 Evaluating Oxygen Saturation and Recognizing Signs of Hypoxia

Oxygen saturation provides a real-time measure of how effectively oxygen is being delivered to the body's tissues. Normal saturation levels typically range between 95% and 100%, while values below 92% are often a sign of hypoxemia that requires immediate intervention. It is essential to understand that oxygen saturation trends are just as important as individual readings, as gradual declines may indicate a worsening condition.

Beyond the numeric value provided by pulse oximetry, nurses must also assess clinical signs of hypoxia. Increased respiratory effort or shortness of breath may be an early indicator, as the body struggles to compensate for reduced oxygen levels. Cyanosis, particularly around the lips or fingertips, is a late and serious sign of oxygen deprivation. Restlessness or confusion may suggest decreased oxygen delivery to the brain, emphasizing the importance of a holistic assessment alongside monitoring tools.

Interventions to address hypoxia depend on the severity of the condition. Adjusting oxygen delivery methods is often the first step, such as increasing the flow rate or transitioning from a nasal cannula to a face mask to provide a higher concentration of oxygen. In more severe cases, non-invasive ventilation or advanced airway management may be required. Ensuring that the client is positioned appropriately—such as sitting upright—can also enhance lung expansion and improve oxygenation.

Documentation is a critical part of this process. Nurses should record the initial oxygen saturation level, the interventions performed, and the client's response. For example, after increasing the oxygen flow rate, it is important to note any improvements in saturation levels or reductions in respiratory distress. Thorough documentation not only provides a clear record for the healthcare team but also ensures continuity of care.

7.4.2 Monitoring Responses to Nasogastric Tube Suction

Nasogastric (NG) tubes are essential for gastric decompression, feeding, or administering medications, but their use requires diligent monitoring to ensure client safety and comfort. Proper oversight of continuous or intermittent suction can help prevent complications such as fluid and electrolyte imbalances, gastric mucosal damage, or tube blockages.

One critical aspect is ensuring that the suction settings are appropriate for the client's condition. Low-intermittent suction is commonly preferred for gastric decompression, as it minimizes the risk of damaging the delicate gastric lining. Nurses should routinely check the suction equipment to confirm that the settings are accurate and functioning correctly. Any irregularities, such as excessive suction or equipment failure, should be addressed promptly to maintain safety.

Monitoring gastric output is equally important. Nurses should document the amount, color, and consistency of the output regularly, as these factors can provide valuable insights into the client's condition. For example, a sudden increase in output volume may indicate unresolved gastric stasis, while the presence of coffee-ground material could signify gastrointestinal bleeding and requires immediate notification of the healthcare provider. Such diligent observation allows for early identification of complications and timely intervention.

Client comfort is another essential consideration. NG tubes can cause irritation and discomfort, manifesting as sore throats, nasal tenderness, or nausea. Regularly assessing for these symptoms and offering comfort measures can significantly improve the client's experience. Suggestions include providing throat lozenges, ensuring proper lubrication of the tube to reduce friction, and encouraging frequent oral hygiene to combat dryness and irritation caused by the tube.

Additionally, nurses should be vigilant for signs of abdominal distension or discomfort, which may indicate a tube blockage or improper functioning. Troubleshooting the issue by flushing the tube with prescribed solutions or adjusting its position can restore its efficacy and alleviate the client's symptoms.

Effective communication with clients is vital throughout the process. Explaining the purpose of the NG tube, suction, and monitoring procedures helps alleviate anxiety and promotes cooperation. In cases where complications arise, clients and families should be informed promptly, along with clear explanations of the steps being taken to resolve the issue.

Chapter 8
Physiological Adaptation

Physiological adaptation focuses on the body's ability to maintain balance and recover from illness or injury. Nurses play a pivotal role in supporting clients as they adapt to changes in their physical health, whether it involves managing chronic conditions, responding to acute illnesses, or assisting with the use of medical devices. This chapter provides a comprehensive guide to recognizing and addressing physiological imbalances, offering evidence-based strategies to optimize client outcomes. Topics include respiratory and cardiac care, wound management, and interventions for clients with fluid, electrolyte, or nutritional challenges. By mastering these concepts, nurses can confidently respond to diverse clinical scenarios, ensuring safety and promoting recovery in all care settings.

8.1 Monitoring and Intervening in Critical Client Conditions

Nurses must remain adept at identifying abnormalities in client presentations, interpreting diagnostic tools, and initiating appropriate interventions to prevent complications and improve outcomes. Key areas of focus include the recognition of cardiac abnormalities, effective responses to emergencies, and early identification of acute or chronic illness.

8.1.1 Recognizing and Reporting Cardiac Abnormalities

Interpreting cardiac monitor strips is a critical skill for identifying potentially life-threatening cardiac abnormalities and ensuring timely intervention. Nurses must be proficient in recognizing dysrhythmias, ischemic changes, and other signs of cardiac distress, as these findings can significantly influence client outcomes.

Familiarity with common dysrhythmias and their implications is essential:

- **Atrial Fibrillation (AFib):** This arrhythmia is characterized by an irregularly irregular rhythm, absent P waves, and fibrillatory waves. AFib increases the risk of thrombus formation, potentially leading to stroke. Management often includes anticoagulation therapy and rate or rhythm control medications.

- **Ventricular Tachycardia (VT):** A life-threatening rhythm identifiable by rapid, wide QRS complexes, VT requires immediate intervention. Depending on the client's condition, interventions may include defibrillation, antiarrhythmic drugs, or advanced cardiac life support (ACLS) protocols.
- **ST-Segment Changes:** Elevation or depression of the ST segment may indicate ischemia or myocardial infarction. Prompt recognition of these changes is vital, as they often require urgent diagnostic or therapeutic measures, such as administering thrombolytics, preparing for cardiac catheterization, or notifying the rapid response team.

To ensure accurate recognition and communication of cardiac abnormalities, nurses should:

- **Monitor Continuously and Document Findings:** Regularly assess monitor strips for changes in rhythm, rate, or waveform morphology. Record essential details, including the date, time, and the nurse's interpretation of the strip.
- **Communicate Promptly:** Notify the healthcare provider immediately upon identifying significant abnormalities, such as sustained VT or signs of ischemia, to facilitate rapid intervention.
- **Correlate with Clinical Symptoms:** Pair findings on the monitor with the client's symptoms. For example, a client experiencing chest pain with ST-segment elevation requires urgent attention, while asymptomatic bradycardia may need closer observation and monitoring.

8.1.2 Responding to Emergencies

Emergencies such as sudden cardiac arrest or acute respiratory failure require immediate, structured responses to preserve life and prevent long-term complications. Nurses play a pivotal role in recognizing these critical events, initiating life-saving interventions, and coordinating care until additional help arrives.

Proficiency in **Basic Life Support (BLS)** and **Cardiopulmonary Resuscitation (CPR)** is essential for managing cardiac emergencies. Key actions include:

- **Airway Management:** Quickly assess and clear the airway to ensure unobstructed oxygen delivery. Techniques may involve head-tilt and chin-lift maneuvers, suctioning, or advanced airway placement in collaboration with the care team.
- **High-Quality Chest Compressions:** Deliver compressions at the recommended depth (2 inches for adults) and rate (100–120 compressions per minute), allowing for full chest recoil to maximize circulation. Consistency and proper hand placement are critical for effective CPR.
- **Defibrillation:** Utilize an **Automated External Defibrillator (AED)** or manual defibrillator for arrhythmias like ventricular fibrillation or pulseless ventricular tachycardia. Follow Advanced Cardiac Life Support (ACLS) protocols, including appropriate drug administration and rhythm monitoring.

In non-cardiac emergencies, such as **acute respiratory distress** or **shock**, rapid assessment and intervention are equally vital:

- **Administer Oxygen:** Initiate supplemental oxygen using the most effective delivery device based on the client's condition, whether through nasal cannula, non-rebreather mask, or bag-valve-mask ventilation.
- **Ensure Venous Access:** Establish intravenous (IV) or intraosseous (IO) access to administer fluids, medications, or blood products promptly. This step is critical in conditions like hypovolemic shock or sepsis.
- **Continuous Monitoring:** Keep a close watch on vital signs and clinical symptoms to evaluate the client's response to interventions. For example, a rising oxygen saturation level or stabilization of blood pressure indicates progress, while worsening signs call for escalated care.

8.1.3 Identifying Early Signs of Acute or Chronic Illness

Early recognition of illness is a cornerstone of effective nursing care, enabling prompt intervention to prevent complications and improve recovery outcomes. Nurses are often the first to observe subtle changes in a client's condition, and their vigilance can make a critical difference in both acute and chronic settings.

In cases of **acute illness**, recognizing key warning signs is essential for initiating life-saving measures. For instance, identifying **sepsis** —a life-threatening systemic infection— requires close attention to symptoms such as:

- **Fever** or **hypothermia**, which may indicate the body's response to infection.
- **Tachycardia** and **hypotension**, early indicators of compromised circulation and systemic inflammation.
- **Altered mental status**, which can suggest reduced oxygen delivery to the brain or the onset of septic shock.

When these signs are present, nurses should act swiftly by following institutional sepsis protocols. This may include obtaining blood cultures, administering broad-spectrum antibiotics, initiating fluid resuscitation, and continuously monitoring vital signs.

In **chronic illness management**, nurses must be attuned to exacerbations that signal worsening conditions. For example, clients with **heart failure** may experience:

- **Increased peripheral edema**, a sign of fluid retention due to poor cardiac output.
- **Sudden weight gain**, often caused by rapid fluid accumulation, which requires adjustments in diuretics or dietary sodium restrictions.
- **Shortness of breath** or fatigue, indicating potential pulmonary congestion or reduced oxygen delivery.

In such scenarios, nurses can help prevent hospital readmissions by identifying these signs early and collaborating with the healthcare team to modify the treatment plan. This might involve titrating medications, reinforcing dietary and fluid management education, or scheduling follow-up care.

8.2 Supporting Respiratory and Ventilatory Function

Maintaining effective respiratory function is crucial for clients with compromised breathing due to acute or chronic conditions. Nurses play a vital role in providing care, monitoring, and interventions for clients requiring respiratory or ventilatory support. This involves managing devices such as tracheostomies and ventilators, as well as employing techniques to improve respiratory status. Expertise in these areas helps prevent complications, promotes client comfort, and enhances outcomes.

8.2.1 Providing Care for Clients with Tracheostomies

Tracheostomy care is a critical component of nursing practice, ensuring that clients with this airway modification maintain optimal respiratory function and avoid complications. Proper care involves a meticulous approach to airway management, stoma maintenance, and client education, all of which contribute to the client's safety, comfort, and long-term well-being.

Suctioning is a fundamental skill for nurses providing tracheostomy care. Clients may exhibit signs of respiratory distress, such as audible secretions, increased respiratory effort, or low oxygen saturation levels. Suctioning helps clear the airway and restore effective breathing. Nurses should:

- Use **sterile technique** to minimize the risk of infection.
- Limit suctioning to **10–15 seconds per pass** and observe the client for signs of distress, such as bradycardia or desaturation.
- Allow **sufficient recovery time** between suctioning attempts to prevent hypoxia and ensure the client's comfort.

Stoma maintenance is equally important in preventing complications such as infection or skin breakdown. Nurses should:

- **Clean the stoma site** regularly using sterile saline and gentle techniques to remove debris and secretions.
- Replace tracheostomy dressings as **needed**, ensuring that the area remains dry and free from moisture, which can promote bacterial growth.
- Monitor the stoma site for **redness, swelling, or discharge**, which may indicate infection. Early detection allows for prompt treatment and reduces the risk of further complications.

Client education is a crucial aspect of tracheostomy care, especially for clients transitioning to home care. Nurses should teach clients and caregivers:

- How to perform daily tracheostomy care, emphasizing the importance of maintaining a **clean environment** to prevent infection.
- The correct technique for suctioning, including how to recognize when it is needed and how to perform it safely.
- Early signs of complications, such as difficulty breathing, persistent redness or swelling around the stoma, or unusual secretions, and the importance of seeking medical attention promptly.

Additionally, clients and their families should feel confident managing the tracheostomy equipment, such as ensuring the availability of spare tracheostomy tubes, suction catheters, and a functioning suction machine in case of emergencies. Nurses can provide hands-on demonstrations and written materials to reinforce learning.

8.2.2 Managing Ventilated Clients

Caring for clients on mechanical ventilation is a critical responsibility that requires vigilant monitoring and proactive interventions to ensure optimal outcomes and prevent complications. Nurses play an essential role in maintaining ventilator function, preventing ventilator-associated pneumonia (VAP), and supporting clients through the weaning and extubation process.

Monitoring Ventilator Settings is a foundational aspect of managing ventilated clients. Nurses must frequently check parameters such as tidal volume, respiratory rate, oxygen concentration, and positive end-expiratory pressure (PEEP) to ensure they align with the healthcare provider's orders and meet the client's needs. Any deviations or alarms, such as high-pressure warnings (which could indicate secretions or tubing obstruction) or low-pressure alarms (suggesting disconnection or leaks), require immediate attention. Nurses should also document ventilator settings and any adjustments made, providing a clear record for the interdisciplinary team.

Preventing Ventilator-Associated Pneumonia (VAP) is a high priority in ventilated client care. VAP is a serious complication that can arise from prolonged mechanical ventilation, often due to bacterial colonization in the respiratory tract. To reduce this risk, nurses should implement evidence-based strategies, including:

- **Head-of-bed elevation:** Keeping the client's head elevated 30–45 degrees reduces the likelihood of aspiration.
- **Oral care:** Providing regular oral hygiene with chlorhexidine not only promotes comfort but also lowers the bacterial load in the oropharyngeal cavity.
- **Closed suction systems:** Using closed systems minimizes exposure to the environment, reducing the risk of infection during suctioning procedures.
- **Sedation protocols:** Evaluating and minimizing sedation levels can encourage spontaneous breathing efforts, which contribute to earlier weaning and reduced VAP risk.

Weaning and Extubation Preparation is an important phase in the care of ventilated clients, requiring close collaboration with the healthcare team. Nurses monitor for indicators of readiness for weaning, such as improved respiratory effort, stable oxygenation levels, and adequate arterial blood gas results. During spontaneous breathing trials, nurses observe the client's ability to maintain oxygenation and ventilation without significant support from the ventilator. Key considerations include:

- **Assessing respiratory effort:** Monitor for signs of fatigue, increased work of breathing, or desaturation, which may signal that the client is not yet ready for extubation.
- **Ensuring adequate support:** Provide reassurance to the client and anticipate needs during weaning trials, such as suctioning to clear secretions or adjusting oxygen delivery.
- **Communicating progress:** Document the client's response to weaning and communicate findings with the healthcare team to guide decisions on extubation timing.

8.2.3 Techniques for Improving Respiratory Status

For clients experiencing respiratory distress, nurses can utilize a variety of evidence-based techniques to enhance breathing and oxygenation. These interventions address airway patency, optimize gas exchange, and support overall respiratory function, tailored to the client's specific condition and needs.

Breathing Treatments are often the first line of intervention for managing respiratory issues such as bronchospasms or inflammation. Administering nebulized medications, like bronchodilators or corticosteroids, can rapidly open airways and reduce inflammation, improving oxygen flow. Nurses should educate clients on proper inhalation techniques, emphasizing slow, deep breaths to ensure the medication reaches the lower airways. For instance, instructing clients to hold their breath briefly after inhalation can maximize medication absorption and therapeutic effect.

Suctioning is critical for removing secretions that obstruct the airways and compromise oxygenation. Whether suctioning the upper airway or using a sterile technique for lower airway suctioning, it is vital to monitor the client closely for any signs of distress. Oxygen saturation should be assessed before, during, and after the procedure to ensure the client remains stable. Limiting suctioning to 10–15 seconds per pass and allowing adequate recovery time between attempts minimizes hypoxia and discomfort. Regular assessment of the client's airway, such as noting gurgling sounds or visible secretions, helps determine the frequency of suctioning.

Repositioning can significantly impact respiratory function by facilitating lung expansion and secretion clearance. Adjusting the client to a semi-Fowler's or high-Fowler's position often alleviates dyspnea and promotes effective diaphragmatic movement. In clients with conditions like acute respiratory distress syndrome (ARDS), prone positioning has been shown to improve oxygenation by redistributing lung perfusion and enhancing ventilation to less compressed lung regions. Nurses should carefully monitor clients during repositioning, observing for changes in oxygen saturation, comfort levels, and respiratory effort.

8.3 Managing Drainage and Wound Care

Proper management of drainage devices and wounds is integral to preventing complications and promoting healing. Nurses are responsible for providing meticulous care for various drainage systems, performing sterile wound care, and assessing wounds for infection or delayed healing. A systematic approach ensures effective treatment and client safety, while promoting comfort and recovery.

8.3.1 Caring for Wound Drains and Chest Tubes

Drainage devices, such as wound drains and chest tubes, play a crucial role in managing postoperative and traumatic conditions by removing excess fluid or air, reducing pressure on surrounding tissues, and promoting healing. Nurses are responsible for maintaining these devices to ensure their functionality and the client's safety.

Wound Drains: Devices like Jackson-Pratt (JP) or Hemovac drains are commonly used after surgical procedures to prevent fluid accumulation that could delay healing or lead to infection. Nurses must regularly empty and measure the output, documenting the volume, color, and consistency. For instance, serosanguineous fluid is a normal finding in the early postoperative period, while purulent or foul-smelling drainage may indicate an infection that requires prompt attention. Nurses should also assess for any blockage in the tubing, which could impede proper drainage and compromise wound healing.

Chest Tubes: These are essential for conditions like pneumothorax or pleural effusion, helping to remove air, blood, or other fluids from the pleural cavity. Nurses should frequently monitor the chest tube system for air leaks, which appear as bubbling in the water seal chamber, and ensure that the system remains at the appropriate level relative to the client to facilitate drainage. Checking the water seal chamber for proper oscillation, known as tidaling, helps confirm that the system is functioning correctly. Assessing the insertion site for infection or subcutaneous emphysema—indicated by a crackling sensation under the skin—ensures early detection of complications. Prompt action, such as notifying the provider or applying appropriate dressings, is crucial for resolving issues.

Device Removal: Removing a wound drain or chest tube requires careful preparation and execution to minimize discomfort and complications. Nurses should follow aseptic techniques, ensuring the area is clean and prepared for removal. Before the procedure, it is important to explain the process to the client, addressing any questions or concerns to reduce anxiety. After removal, closely monitor the client for excessive bleeding, changes in respiratory status (for chest tubes), or signs of inadequate drainage that could require further intervention.

8.3.2 Performing Wound Care and Sterile Dressing Changes

Wound care is a vital nursing responsibility that requires strict adherence to sterile techniques to minimize the risk of infection and promote optimal healing. Each wound has unique characteristics, and nurses must assess and tailor their approach based on the type, severity, and underlying cause of the wound.

Sterile Dressing Changes: Conducting sterile dressing changes is essential to protecting the wound from contamination while supporting the healing process. Before beginning, nurses must prepare a sterile field and use sterile gloves and supplies to clean the wound thoroughly. This often includes irrigating the wound with saline or other prescribed solutions to remove debris or exudate. Applying prescribed topical agents, such as antimicrobial ointments or specialized dressings, ensures that the wound remains protected and facilitates the regeneration of healthy tissue. Nurses should document key observations, such as the wound's size, depth, color, presence of granulation tissue, and the type and amount of exudate. For example, clear or slightly yellow fluid may be normal, whereas thick, green, or foul-smelling drainage could indicate infection.

Suture or Staple Removal: Removing sutures or staples is a precise process that requires close assessment of the wound's condition. The provider's timeline for removal is critical to ensure the wound edges have adequately healed and are no longer at risk of reopening. Using sterile tools, nurses carefully remove each suture or staple while monitoring the client for discomfort and checking for signs of wound separation. After removal, applying steri-strips or other supportive measures may be necessary to maintain the integrity of the wound. Nurses must also assess for redness, swelling, or other signs of delayed healing that might require additional intervention.

Client Education: Empowering clients to care for their wounds at home is a key component of the recovery process. Nurses should provide clear instructions on maintaining hygiene, performing dressing changes, and applying any prescribed medications. Clients must also be taught to recognize early signs of complications, such as increased redness, warmth, swelling, or drainage, and to seek medical attention promptly if these occur. For example, a client recovering from surgery may be advised to keep the wound dry during bathing, change dressings daily, and avoid strenuous activities that could disrupt the healing process.

8.3.3 Assessing Wounds for Infection or Delayed Healing

Regular and thorough assessment of wounds is a critical nursing responsibility to ensure timely identification and management of potential complications. Early recognition of issues such as infection or delayed healing can significantly improve outcomes by enabling prompt interventions.

Signs of Infection: Nurses must be vigilant in detecting local and systemic indicators of infection. Locally, wounds exhibiting redness, warmth, swelling, purulent or foul-smelling drainage, and increased tenderness are likely to be infected. These signs may be accompanied by systemic symptoms, such as fever, chills, or an elevated white blood cell count, which could suggest the infection has spread. For example, a client presenting with a wound that produces greenish, malodorous exudate and displays surrounding erythema may require immediate wound culture and antibiotic therapy to prevent further complications.

Healing Progress: Effective wound care involves monitoring the wound's progression over time. Positive indicators, such as the presence of healthy granulation tissue, a reduction in wound size, and minimal, clear exudate, suggest proper healing. However, delayed healing—evidenced by persistent size, excessive drainage, or a lack of granulation tissue—can be linked to underlying factors like poor circulation, diabetes, or malnutrition. For instance, a client with diabetes might exhibit slowed healing due to impaired blood flow and increased susceptibility to infection.

Interventions: When complications arise, a collaborative approach is crucial. For infected wounds, nurses may assist in obtaining wound cultures and administering prescribed antibiotics. Adjustments to the wound care plan, such as changing dressings more frequently or incorporating antimicrobial agents, may also be necessary. In cases of delayed healing, introducing advanced wound care strategies like negative pressure wound therapy (NPWT) can enhance tissue regeneration by promoting blood flow and reducing edema. Additionally, nurses should work with dietitians to address nutritional deficits, such as insufficient protein or vitamin C, which are essential for wound healing.

8.4 Maintaining Fluid and Electrolyte Balance

Maintaining fluid and electrolyte balance is essential for homeostasis and optimal physiological function. Imbalances can lead to serious complications, particularly in clients with chronic conditions or those undergoing treatments like dialysis. Nurses play a critical role in identifying, addressing, and educating clients about fluid and electrolyte management to ensure stability and prevent further health issues.

8.4.1 Recognizing and Managing Imbalances

Fluid and electrolyte imbalances are common yet critical conditions that require vigilant monitoring and timely intervention. These imbalances can significantly impact various body systems, particularly the cardiovascular, neurological, and renal systems. Nurses play a pivotal role in recognizing early signs and managing these conditions effectively.

Dehydration: Dehydration often manifests through symptoms such as dry mucous membranes, decreased skin turgor, hypotension, tachycardia, and concentrated urine. Clients experiencing mild dehydration may benefit from oral rehydration solutions, while severe cases often necessitate intravenous fluids to restore fluid balance quickly. Monitoring the client's weight, urine output, and electrolyte levels is essential to gauge the effectiveness of interventions. For example, a client presenting with confusion and tachycardia after prolonged vomiting may require both fluid replacement and electrolyte correction.

Fluid Overload: Fluid retention, often associated with conditions like heart failure or kidney dysfunction, can lead to symptoms such as peripheral or pulmonary edema, shortness of breath, and elevated blood pressure. Interventions may include fluid restriction, administration of prescribed diuretics, and positioning the client with their head elevated to improve respiratory function. For instance, a client with visible ankle edema and dyspnea might benefit from furosemide administration, coupled with ongoing monitoring of their weight and respiratory status.

Electrolyte Imbalances: Imbalances in key electrolytes like potassium, sodium, and calcium can cause serious complications, particularly affecting the neuromuscular and cardiac systems:

- **Hyperkalemia:** Elevated potassium levels can result in muscle weakness, paresthesia, and life-threatening arrhythmias. Treatments such as Kayexalate, insulin with glucose, or emergency dialysis may be needed, depending on the severity.
- **Hyponatremia:** Low sodium levels can cause symptoms ranging from lethargy to seizures. Treatment focuses on cautious sodium replacement, typically through oral supplements or IV saline, while addressing the underlying cause, such as fluid overload or excessive diuretic use.
- **Hypocalcemia:** This imbalance often presents as muscle spasms, tetany, or tingling around the mouth and extremities. Correcting calcium levels through dietary changes, IV calcium gluconate, or supplementation helps alleviate these symptoms and prevent complications.

Regular laboratory monitoring is essential for tracking trends in fluid and electrolyte levels, particularly for clients with chronic illnesses or those receiving treatments like diuretics or dialysis. Nurses should perform frequent assessments, including evaluating cardiac rhythm, neurological status, and fluid balance indicators like weight and urine output.

8.4.2 Caring for Clients Undergoing Peritoneal or Hemodialysis

Dialysis is a critical intervention for managing end-stage renal disease (ESRD) or acute kidney failure, enabling clients to maintain fluid and electrolyte balance and remove waste products from the body. The nurse's role in dialysis care is multifaceted, encompassing preparation, monitoring, and post-procedure care to ensure the safety and well-being of the client.

Peritoneal Dialysis: This form of dialysis involves infusing dialysate into the peritoneal cavity, where it absorbs waste products and excess fluids before being drained. Nurses must carefully monitor the infusion and drainage process to ensure proper flow and detect any complications:

- **Effluent Assessment:** The clarity of the drained fluid is a critical indicator of peritoneal health. Cloudy effluent can signal peritonitis, a potentially life-threatening infection. Nurses should promptly report such findings, and clients may require immediate antibiotic therapy.
- **Catheter Care:** The peritoneal catheter site should be monitored for signs of infection, such as redness, swelling, or discharge. Adhering to strict sterile technique during exchanges and dressing changes minimizes the risk of infection.

- **Client Comfort:** Clients may experience discomfort during the process. Nurses should ensure that the dialysate is warmed to body temperature before infusion and encourage clients to report any abdominal pain or bloating.

Hemodialysis: This procedure involves filtering the client's blood through a machine to remove toxins, excess fluids, and electrolytes. Nurses play a key role in ensuring the process runs smoothly and safely:

- **Monitoring During Dialysis:** Clients undergoing hemodialysis are at risk for complications such as hypotension, muscle cramps, or dizziness due to fluid shifts. Nurses should monitor vital signs closely and provide interventions, such as adjusting fluid removal rates or administering prescribed medications, to alleviate symptoms.
- **Vascular Access Care:** The functionality and integrity of the vascular access site, whether an arteriovenous (AV) fistula, graft, or central line, must be evaluated regularly. Nurses should assess for the presence of a bruit and thrill, indicating patency, and inspect for signs of infection, such as redness or swelling.

Client Monitoring and Post-Dialysis Care:

- **Pre- and Post-Dialysis Assessments:** Nurses should assess the client's weight, blood pressure, and fluid balance before and after dialysis to evaluate the procedure's effectiveness. Notable weight changes can reflect the amount of fluid removed during treatment.
- **Electrolyte Monitoring:** Blood samples may be taken to measure levels of potassium, calcium, and other electrolytes. Results guide adjustments in dialysate composition or medications.
- **Client Education:** Teach clients about self-care, such as protecting their vascular access site, recognizing signs of complications, and adhering to dietary and fluid restrictions to optimize dialysis outcomes.

8.4.3 Educating Clients on Fluid and Electrolyte Management

Educating clients about fluid and electrolyte management is crucial, particularly for those with chronic conditions like heart failure, kidney disease, or hypertension, where imbalances can exacerbate symptoms or lead to severe complications. Nurses play a pivotal role in providing clients with practical, clear guidance to help them maintain optimal health and prevent avoidable emergencies.

Fluid Intake Management: Clients must understand the importance of regulating their fluid intake to prevent issues like dehydration or fluid overload. This is especially vital for those on fluid restrictions due to conditions such as chronic kidney disease or heart failure. Nurses should:

- Teach clients how to measure and track their daily fluid consumption accurately. Suggest simple tools, like a designated container or diary, to make monitoring manageable.

- Offer strategies for managing thirst, which can be particularly challenging for those on restricted intake. Tips like sipping fluids slowly, sucking on ice chips, or chewing sugar-free gum can help alleviate discomfort without exceeding limits.

Recognizing Symptoms of Imbalances: Clients should be educated on the signs of both fluid and electrolyte imbalances, empowering them to seek help promptly when needed. For example:

- **Signs of Dehydration:** Dry mouth, decreased skin elasticity, dark urine, and dizziness.
- **Signs of Fluid Overload:** Swelling in the extremities, shortness of breath, or sudden weight gain.
- **Electrolyte Imbalances:** Muscle cramps, irregular heartbeats, confusion, or tingling sensations. Encourage clients to monitor themselves regularly and report any concerning symptoms to their healthcare provider without delay.

Dietary Guidance: A tailored approach to diet can significantly impact fluid and electrolyte balance. Nurses should provide personalized recommendations that align with the client's condition:

- **Sodium Restriction:** For clients prone to fluid retention, emphasize reducing sodium intake by avoiding processed foods, canned goods, and high-sodium seasonings. Encourage the use of herbs and spices to enhance flavor without adding salt.
- **Potassium-Rich Foods:** Clients with hypokalemia should be guided to include potassium-rich options such as bananas, oranges, spinach, and sweet potatoes in their diet, unless contraindicated by a condition like kidney failure.
- **Phosphorus and Calcium:** Educate clients with chronic kidney disease about managing phosphorus and calcium levels to prevent bone complications, advising on appropriate food choices and the use of prescribed binders if needed.

QUESTION BANK

1. During a nutritional class for patients considering weight loss surgery, a 30-year-old female client asks about dietary changes post-surgery. What should the nurse emphasize as the most critical aspect of post-operative nutrition?

   [A] Consuming protein-rich foods is essential for recovery

   [B] You should focus on liquid diets immediately after surgery

   [C] Eating larger meals will help with your energy levels

   [D] You'll need to avoid all carbohydrates completely

2. What is the recommended administration method for furosemide (Lasix) IV in a client with severe hypertension?

   [A] By administering it as a continuous infusion

   [B] By using an infusion pump

   [C] By mixing with dextrose solution

   [D] By administering it through a venous access device

3. For a client experiencing frequent choking episodes while eating, which intervention is essential to consider?

   [A] Encouraging the client to eat quickly

   [B] Providing a diet of only solid foods

   [C] Tilting the head back during swallowing

   [D] Implementing thicker food textures in the diet

4. What criminal charge could result from a nursing graduate practicing under a title they have not been licensed for?

   [A] Fraud

   [B] Assault

   [C] Battery

   [D] Theft

5. What is an important consideration when administering furosemide (Lasix) IV to a patient with acute hypertension?

   [A] To give it rapidly to lower blood pressure quickly

   [B] To administer it at a rate of approximately 1 mL per minute

   [C] To dilute it with sterile water

   [D] To mix it with potassium chloride

6. What laboratory finding should the nurse monitor in a patient taking phenytoin (Dilantin) for seizure management that could indicate toxicity?

[A] Liver function tests elevated

[B] Serum electrolytes normal

[C] Urinalysis negative for ketones

[D] Plasma phenytoin level of 25 mcg/mL

7. When caring for an infant with Hemophilia, which aspect should a nurse prioritize to promote healthy emotional development?

[A] Physical rehabilitation exercises

[B] Individualized care plans

[C] Supportive family interactions

[D] Minimizing medical interventions

8. When caring for an avulsed tooth, the client should be instructed to avoid contact with which part of the tooth?

[A] The enamel

[B] The root

[C] The crown

[D] The gum line

9. What type of burn typically causes blisters and is characterized by intense pain?

[A] First degree burn

[B] Third degree burn

[C] Second degree burn

[D] Fourth degree burn

10. After a change of shift report, which client should the nurse assess first?

[A] A client with a temperature of 101.5°F after abdominal surgery

[B] A client with a feeding tube who is stable

[C] A client with mild dehydration who is alert

[D] A client with chest tube drainage of 50 cc who is in respiratory distress

11. Which electrolyte is primarily responsible for regulating fluid balance in the body?

[A] Potassium

[B] Sodium

[C] Calcium

[D] Magnesium

12. Which of the following practices regarding umbilical cord care is considered appropriate and does not require further instruction?

[A] Applying ointment to the cord to prevent infection

[B] Covering the cord with a tight-fitting diaper

[C] Keeping the cord clean and dry by washing hands before and after care

[D] Bathing the newborn immediately after birth

13. A patient requires 800 cc of IV fluid to be infused over 6 hours using a drip set that delivers 10 cc/drop. Calculate the infusion rate in gtts/min.

[A] 22.2 gtts/min

[B] 25 gtts/min

[B] 30 gtts/min

[D] 40 gtts/min

14. What technique should a nurse recommend to a patient with dysphagia to help prevent aspiration during meals?

[A] Swallowing with the head tilted to the side

[B] Tucking the chin towards the chest while swallowing

[C] Taking smaller bites of food

[D] Using a straw for drinking liquids

15. After a mastectomy, which of the following activities is advised first for rehabilitation?

[A] Doing push-ups

[B] Jogging

[C] Ball squeezing exercises

[D] Rotating the shoulder

16. In which condition is it important to monitor uric acid levels?

[A] Gout

[B] Hypertension

[C] Diabetes

[D] Anemia

17. Which of the following factors increases the likelihood of having twins?

[A] Low maternal age

[B] Single pregnancies

[C] Smoking during pregnancy

[D] Advanced maternal age

18. A nurse caring for which of the following clients should exercise caution due to potential radiation exposure?

[A] The client receiving chemotherapy for leukemia

[B] The client who has just undergone surgery for lung cancer

[C] The client with a sealed radioactive implant for breast cancer

[D] The client admitted for observation after a CT scan

19. Which of the following cancers is known for developing in the liver and primarily affects young children?

[A] Nephroblastoma

[B] Brain cancer

[C] Basal cell carcinoma

[D] Hepatoblastoma

20. Which of the following measures is most effective for a patient with liver disease experiencing pruritus?

[A] Add oatmeal to the bath water

[B] Recommend excessive sun exposure for vitamin D

[C] Suggest using a thick, fragrance-free lotion after bathing

[D] Instruct to use hot water during baths

21. Which of the following is true regarding mammography for women with breast implants?

[A] It requires specialized imaging techniques

[B] Implants are a common contraindication for the procedure

[C] It cannot be performed after surgery

[D] It involves less radiation exposure

22. What is the primary cause of Cushing's syndrome?

[A] Underproduction of thyroid hormones

[B] Overproduction of insulin by the pancreas

[C] Lack of adrenal glands function

[D] Overproduction of cortisol by the adrenal glands

23. What type of joint allows for rotational movement and has the greatest range of motion?

[A] Ball-and-socket joint

[B] Hinge joint

[C] Pivot joint

[D] Saddle joint

24. A patient diagnosed with pancreatitis is experiencing severe abdominal pain. What intervention should the nurse prioritize?

[A] Starting a catheterization

[B] Administering IV fluids

[C] Assisting with ambulation

[D] Performing wound care

25. Which client would be the most appropriate for shared accommodation with a patient diagnosed with myasthenia gravis?

[A] A client recovering from surgery

[B] A client with diabetes

[C] A client with hypothyroidism

[D] A client with heart failure

26. During a wellness check, a nurse notes that a patient is 52 years old and has not had a menstrual period in over a year. What phase of life is this patient likely experiencing?

[A] Menopause

[B] Perimenopause

[C] Climacteric

[D] Premenstrual syndrome

27. What is the primary characteristic of the congenital heart defect known as Tetralogy of Fallot?

[A] It primarily affects the lungs

[B] It consists of four heart defects

[C] It is associated with digestive issues

[D] It is caused by viral infections

28. Lidocaine is commonly administered to manage which cardiac condition?

[A] Atrial fibrillation

[B] Supraventricular tachycardia

[C] Myocardial infarction

[D] Ventricular tachycardia

29. In a trauma situation, which assessment finding should alert the nurse to possible respiratory distress?

[A] Decreased blood pressure

[B] Stridor

[C] Increased heart rate

[D] Edema of the limbs

30. Which condition may indicate the need for immediate intervention in a patient with hepatic insufficiency?

[A] Dehydration

[B] Constipation

[C] Insomnia

[D] Coma

31. Which symptom would indicate a nurse to reassess the appropriateness of hormone replacement therapy in a menopausal patient?

[A] Family history of breast cancer

[B] Unexplained vaginal bleeding

[C] Increased libido

[D] Mood swings

32. Which of the following is an unlikely manifestation in a client diagnosed with laryngeal cancer?

[A] Weight loss

[B] Frequent throat clearing

[C] Severe headaches

[D] Voice changes

33. What should a nurse do if the dialysate from a patient undergoing peritoneal dialysis appears cloudy?

[A] Send a specimen to the lab

[B] Administer additional dialysis

[C] Document the finding

[D] Increase the dialysate volume

34. Which term describes the discharge from a wound that is thin and red, often present in surgical wounds?

[A] Purulent

[B] Sanguinous

[C] Serosanguineous

[D] Necrotic

35. For an 18-month-old child, which of the following activities is considered developmentally appropriate?

[A] Playing with a soft stuffed animal

[B] Completing a coloring book

[C] Using scissors for craft

[D] Playing complex board games

36. A patient with hepatic disease is experiencing severe itching. What is the best nursing intervention to relieve this symptom?

[A] Advise the patient to use harsh soaps

[B] Instruct the patient to add mineral oil to their bath

[C] Encourage the patient to take long, hot showers

[D] Suggest the use of alcohol-based lotions

37. During the preoperative assessment of a patient with an aortic aneurysm, which finding should the nurse prioritize?

[A] Arranging transportation for the patient post-surgery

[B] Evaluating the presence of peripheral pulse

[C] Reviewing the patient's medication list

[D] Confirming the patient's allergies

38. When evaluating a patient for a suspected myocardial infarction, which test is less specific than other cardiac biomarkers?

[A] Troponin

[B] CK-MB

[C] AST

[D] Myoglobin

39. Which of the following can act as a vector for spreading diseases?

[A] A used syringe

[B] A contaminated water source

[C] A mosquito

[D] A soap bar

40. Which medication is commonly used to manage symptoms of Meniere's disease?

[A] Antivert

[B] Lisinopril

[C] Metformin

[D] Simvastatin

41. What is a potential challenge of performing a mammogram on a patient with breast implants?

[A] They might obscure the visualization of breast tissue

[B] They are not safe for mammography

[C] They can cause an allergic reaction to contrast

[D] They increase radiation exposure

42. When educating a patient about the potential side effects of chemotherapy for Hodgkin's disease, which adverse effect should the nurse highlight that could lead to feelings of altered body image?

[A] Nausea

[B] Fatigue

[C] Decreased libido

[D] Alopecia

43. At what age is it generally recommended to perform surgical correction for a cleft palate in infants?

[A] 20 to 24 months of age

[B] 8 to 12 months of age

[C] 16 to 20 months of age

[D] 12 to 16 months of age

44. Which personal protective equipment is minimally required for airborne transmission precautions?

[A] Surgical mask

[B] Face shield

[C] Negative pressure room

[D] Gloves

45. Which intervention can help prevent periwound maceration?

[A] Applying tape directly to the wound

[B] Using saline for cleaning the wound

[C] Choosing the appropriate dressing for the wound type

[D] Allowing the wound to remain uncovered

46. Which diagnostic test is commonly used to assess breast abnormalities?

[A] CT scan

[B] MRI

[C] X-ray

[D] Mammogram

47. What condition is characterized by severe weight loss and muscle wasting due to chronic illness?

[A] Cachexia

[B] Anorexia

[C] Malnutrition

[D] Dehydration

48. Which of the following statements is true regarding the use of lactulose in patients with hepatic encephalopathy?

[A] It helps increase blood pressure

[B] It binds to potassium in the intestines

[C] It promotes the absorption of nutrients

[D] It decreases ammonia absorption in the gut

49. Which condition is characterized by progressive muscle weakness and is often mistakenly attributed to normal developmental delays?

[A] Osteomyelitis

[B] Talipes

[C] Duchenne's muscular dystrophy

[D] Septic arthritis

50. What should the nurse do when a client scheduled for surgery does not understand the procedure and its risks?

[A] Provide the client with a pamphlet about the surgery

[B] Reassure the client that everything will be fine

[C] Contact the surgeon to discuss the procedure with the client

[D] Refer the client to a social worker for further assistance

51. When caring for a patient with xerostomia, which option is best to enhance oral comfort?

[A] Offering mouthwash with alcohol

[B] Using a saliva substitute

[C] Encouraging spicy foods

[D] Recommending caffeinated drinks

52. What is the correct order of stages in the infection process?

[A] Illness, convalescence, inflammation, incubation

[B] Incubation, prodromal, illness, and convalescence

[C] Recovery, acute, and prodromal stages

[D] Convalescence, incubation, and primary stages

53. Which nursing action is essential for managing an infant with physiologic jaundice effectively?

[A] Encourage hydration through oral fluids

[B] Avoid any tactile stimulation

[C] Use dark clothing to keep the baby warm

[D] Limit feeding to every 4 hours

54. What term describes a localized collection of blood between the fetal skull and the periosteum that does not cross suture lines?

[A] Caput succedaneum

[B] Molding

[C] Cephalohematoma

[D] Subdural hematoma

55. A patient undergoing chemotherapy presents with lab results indicating a potassium level of 2.5 mEq/L. What condition is this patient likely experiencing?

[A] Hyponatremia

[B] Hyperkalemia

[C] Thrombocytopenia

[D] Hypokalemia

56. What is the daily caloric requirement for a full-term infant aged 1-2 months?

[A] 120 calories per kilogram per day

[B] 100 calories per kilogram per day

[C] 140 calories per kilogram per day

[D] 160 calories per kilogram per day

57. Which practice is most effective for minimizing the risk of healthcare-associated infections?

[A] Using gloves when necessary

[B] Wearing a mask during procedures

[C] Sterilizing instruments properly

[D] Performing hand hygiene regularly

58. Which category of risk factors includes lifestyle choices such as smoking and substance abuse?

[A] Psychosocial

[B] Environmental

[C] Biophysical

[D] Social demographic

59. What is a potential risk for women who breastfeed for extended periods?

[A] Weight gain

[B] Osteoporosis

[C] Excessive milk production

[D] Allergic reactions in infants

60. Which technique uses electronic devices to assist patients in managing their stress responses and physiological activity?

[A] Biofeedback

[B] Guided imagery

[C] Hypnosis

[D] Breathing exercises

61. During the administration of TPN, which lab result indicates a risk for complications due to carbohydrate infusion?

[A] Hemoglobin

[B] Blood glucose

[C] Blood urea nitrogen

[D] Serum calcium

62. What describes the breath sounds that are expected in a patient with clear lung disclosures?

[A] Vesicular breath sounds

[B] Coarse rales

[C] Stridor

[D] Crackles

63. What effect does immobility have on a patient's nitrogen balance?

[A] Negative nitrogen balance

[B] Positive nitrogen balance

[C] No effect on nitrogen balance

[D] Increases protein synthesis

64. Who proposed the stages of psychosocial development throughout the lifespan?

[A] Freud

[B] Erikson

[C] Maslow

[D] Bandura

65. What should a charge nurse do if a staff nurse is suspected of falsifying patient records?

[A] Issue a verbal warning

[B] Create a performance improvement plan

[C] Document the incident and file a formal reprimand

[D] Report to the police

66. What should a nurse do if they observe unprofessional behavior in a care team member interacting with a patient?

[A] Report the incident to hospital administration

[B] Ignore the behavior, as it is not their place to intervene

[C] Discuss the behavior with the care team member privately

[D] Document the incident in the patient's chart

67. A client experiences evisceration of a surgical wound after coughing. What is the best immediate nursing intervention?

[A] Notify the surgeon immediately

[B] Reinsert the organ back into the abdomen

[C] Apply a non-sterile dressing over the wound

[D] Cover the exposed organs with a sterile saline-soaked dressing

68. What is a key requirement for obtaining a practical nursing license?

[A] Passing the NCLEX-PN examination

[B] Completing a nursing certification program

[C] Obtaining a bachelor's degree in nursing

[D] Being a member of a professional nursing organization

69. What lifestyle factor is commonly associated with a higher risk of deep vein thrombosis?

[A] Sedentary behavior

[B] Regular exercise

[C] Prolonged immobility

[D] High protein diet

70. What is the typical composition of an infant's skull in terms of bony structure?

[A] 7

[B] 3

[C] 5

[D] 6

71. Which level of consciousness indicates the least response to stimuli?

[A] Comatose

[B] Lethargic

[C] Alert

[D] Confused

72. What document expresses a patient's wishes regarding specific medical treatments they do not wish to receive?

[A] Durable power of attorney

[B] Advance directives

[C] Healthcare surrogate

[D] Healthcare proxy

73. Which type of cast is preferred to manage swelling and prevent complications like compartment syndrome?

[A] A solid plaster cast for stability

[B] A bivalve cast for pressure relief

[C] A fiberglass cast for quick drying

[D] A removable splint for easier access

74. Which formula is primarily used to calculate fluid resuscitation needs in burn patients?

[A] Lund and Browder chart

[B] Rule of Nines

[C] Parkland Formula

[D] Rule of Tens

75. What type of incident is a power outage in a healthcare facility classified as?

[A] An external disaster

[B] A minor incident

[C] A routine event

[D] An internal disaster

76. In which client should the home health nurse assess for potential complications first?

[A] A client managing obesity with a diet plan

[B] A client with asthma who reports wheezing

[C] A client with hypertension regularly taking medications

[D] A client with arthritis experiencing joint pain

77. Which laboratory test is least useful for confirming a diagnosis of myocardial infarction?

[A] AST

[B] Troponin

[C] CK-MB

[D] Myoglobin

78. A nurse is explaining the typical weight changes in newborns. What is a normal explanation for initial weight loss?

[A] The baby is not feeding well and is losing nutrients

[B] The baby is losing weight due to a metabolic disorder

[C] The baby may lose up to 10% of their birth weight due to fluid loss and meconium passage

[D] The baby is experiencing an adverse reaction to vaccinations

79. Which nurse is most qualified to monitor a client experiencing hypertension during the postpartum period?

[A] The nurse with 1 year of experience in maternal health

[B] The nurse with 4 years of experience in obstetrics

[C] The nurse with 5 years of experience in pediatrics

[D] The nurse with 2 years of experience in surgical care

80. During a disaster drill, which client should receive priority treatment based on their condition?

[A] A child with a headache

[B] An adult with a broken toe

[C] An elderly person with a fever

[D] A young adult with respiratory distress

81. What type of fat should a patient with hyperlipidemia limit in their diet?

[A] Polyunsaturated fat

[B] Monounsaturated fat

[C] Omega-3 fatty acids

[D] Saturated fat

82. Which situation requires immediate notification to the state Board of Nursing?

[A] A nurse fails to execute a physician's orders for a client with a critical condition

[B] A patient is unhappy with the care they received

[C] A patient reports feeling anxious before a procedure

[D] A nurse does not wash hands before caring for a patient with an infectious disease

83. What is the correct order of levels of consciousness, ranked from most to least responsive?

[A] Confused

[B] Stuporous

[C] Alert

[D] Comatose

84. Which stage of anesthesia is characterized by a decreased response to stimuli and is typically safe for surgical procedures?

[A] Stage I

[B] Stage II

[C] Stage III

[D] Stage IV

85. Which condition is characterized by a patient requiring higher doses of medication to achieve the same pain relief?

[A] Drug addiction

[B] Drug interactions

[C] Drug side effects

[D] Drug tolerance

86. Which demographic is more likely to develop appendicitis?

[A] Individuals over the age of 60

[B] Children under the age of 5

[C] Pregnant women

[D] Teenagers and young adults

87. What is the initial recommended exercise for a client recovering from a mastectomy?

[A] Lifting weights

[B] Swimming

[C] Squeezing a soft ball

[D] Stretching arms overhead

88. Which condition is most likely to cause elevated intracranial pressure leading to papilledema?

[A] Severe dehydration

[B] Chronic hypertension

[C] Brain tumor

[D] Migraine headache

89. How many minims are there in 5 milliliters?

[A] 80

[B] 100

[C] 120

[D] 60

90. What factor is most likely to correlate with the psychosocial development of an infant diagnosed with a chronic condition like Hemophilia?

[A] Limited social interaction

[B] Frequent hospitalizations

[C] Physical activity limitations

[D] Changes in family dynamics

91. Which individual has the highest risk of developing gallstones due to common demographic risk factors?

[A] A 60-year-old male patient with diabetes

[B] A 70-year-old female patient with gallbladder disease

[C] A 40-year-old female patient who is Hispanic

[D] A 50-year-old male patient with obesity

92. Which of the following is a characteristic of adjuvant medication for pain management?

[A] They are only used in patients with cancer

[B] They enhance the efficacy of primary analgesics

[C] They are only prescribed after surgery

[D] They must always be administered intravenously

93. Which type of breath sound is typically heard in healthy lungs and indicates normal airflow?

[A] Wheezes

[B] Rhonchi

[C] Fine rales

[D] Vesicular breath sounds

94. Which condition is associated with a lack of antidiuretic hormone?

[A] Diabetes mellitus

[B] Diabetes insipidus

[C] Syndrome of inappropriate antidiuretic hormone

[D] Addison's disease

95. What is a characteristic feature of a Stage IV pressure ulcer?

[A] Exposure of bone, muscle, or tendons

[B] Partial thickness loss of skin

[C] Presence of intact skin

[D] Blanchable erythema

96. What is the most appropriate expected outcome for a patient recovering from surgery related to pain management?

[A] The patient will express satisfaction with pain relief

[B] The nurse will evaluate the patient's pain level every shift

[C] The patient will rate their pain as 3 or less on a scale of 0 to 10

[D] The nurse will teach the patient about pain medications

97. A client expresses a wish to have a spiritual leader present during surgery for support. What is the best response by the nurse?

[A] Surgery is too serious for spiritual beliefs

[B] I will help you arrange for your spiritual leader to be present

[C] That is not necessary for medical care

[D] We cannot accommodate personal beliefs in the operating room

98. Which task is outside the scope of practice for a licensed practical nurse?

[A] Assisting in the insertion of a central line

[B] Administering a blood transfusion

[C] Monitoring vital signs

[D] Providing wound care

99. Which dietary recommendation should be made for a client with osteoporosis?

[A] Increase caffeine intake for improved bone health

[B] Include sources of calcium and vitamin D in the diet

[C] Reduce protein intake to avoid calcium loss

[D] Limit all dairy products as they can harm bone density

100. Which assessment technique should a nurse use to evaluate the presence of an irregular heart rate?

[A] Apical pulse assessment

[B] Capillary refill test

[C] Skin turgor assessment

[D] Bowel sounds auscultation

101. Which hormone is primarily responsible for initiating lactation in new mothers?

[A] Oxytocin

[B] Prolactin

[C] Luteinizing hormone

[D] Follicle-stimulating hormone

102. When providing post-mortem care to a deceased patient, which of the following actions is required?

[A] Only wearing a mask and gloves

[B] Place the patient in a sealed container

[C] Bathe the patient using standard precautions

[D] Leave the body undisturbed

103. Which client would benefit most from being admitted to a medical unit specializing in mental health?

[A] A 30-year-old female recovering from a hip replacement

[B] A 28-year-old female experiencing a manic episode

[C] A 45-year-old male with diabetes mellitus

[D] A 60-year-old male with abdominal pain

104. What term describes the gradual opening of the cervix during labor?

[A] Effacement

[B] Symphysis

[C] Hyperplasia

[D] Dilation

105. What condition is closely related to the development of Osgood-Schlatter disease?

[A] Tendinitis in the elbow

[B] Stress fractures in the foot

[C] Patellar tendon inflammation due to repetitive stress

[D] Bursitis of the shoulder

106. Which nursing theorist is known for the Self-Care Deficit Theory?

[A] Dorothea Orem

[B] Madeleine Leininger

[C] Martha Rogers

[D] Sister Callista Roy

107. What is a safe and effective approach to manage constipation in pregnant individuals?

[A] Taking strong prescription laxatives

[B] Reducing activity levels and resting

[C] Lying flat on the stomach

[D] Increasing water intake and dietary fiber

108. A 48-year-old woman reports experiencing hot flashes and mood swings. The nurse recognizes these symptoms are typical of which phase in a woman's reproductive life?

[A] Menopause

[B] Postmenopause

[C] Perimenopause

[D] Climacteric

109. Identify the type of fracture characterized by a bone that breaks incompletely, often seen in children.

[A] A complete fracture: breaks the bone into two or more pieces

[B] A greenstick fracture: bends and partially breaks the bone

[C] A spiral fracture: occurs due to a twisting force

[D] An avulsion fracture: where a fragment of bone is pulled away

110. Which theorist is known for the theory of moral development?

[A] Bowlby

[B] Kohlberg

[C] Vygotsky

[D] Skinner

111. Which assessment is typically performed to evaluate kidney function during prenatal care?

[A] Blood pressure measurement

[B] Fetal heart rate monitoring

[C] Pelvic examination

[D] Urinalysis for proteins and glucose

112. Which of the following best describes an episiotomy?

[A] A procedure to administer anesthesia

[B] A surgical incision in the perineum during delivery

[C] An incision made in the abdomen for delivery

[D] A step taken to clamp the umbilical cord

113. Which scenario best describes a patient at risk for a healthcare-acquired infection?

[A] A 55-year-old female with an indwelling urinary catheter

[B] A 30-year-old male with a recent cold

[C] A 73-year-old female with no current health issues

[D] A 60-year-old male admitted for elective surgery without any invasive devices

114. After a client has undergone surgery for a pituitary tumor, which of the following findings would prompt immediate intervention by the nurse?

[A] Mild headache

[B] Increased appetite

[C] Elevated blood pressure

[D] Clear drainage from the nose

115. What is a critical instruction for a patient being discharged with an implantable cardioverter-defibrillator (ICD)?

[A] Avoid using phones on the side of the ICD

[B] You can swim immediately after discharge

[C] It's safe to live near high-voltage power lines

[D] You may resume normal activities without restrictions

116. What does the acronym ABCDE refer to in evaluating a patient's health risks preoperatively?

[A] Allergy, bleeding, cortisone, diabetes, emboli

[B] Allergy, brain, cardio, digestive, endocrine

[C] Anxiety, bleeding, cardiovascular, diabetes, edema

[D] Allergy, bleeding, circulatory, diet, environment

117. What is the term for the period of pregnancy from fertilization until the end of the 12th week?

[A] Fetal period

[B] Neonatal period

[C] Labor stage

[D] Embryonic period

118. What is the primary focus of evidence-based practice in nursing?

[A] Using the best available research to guide patient care

[B] Implementing practices based solely on tradition

[C] Following institutional protocols without question

[D] Relying on expert opinion alone

119. Which food item should a client with diverticulitis avoid to minimize abdominal discomfort?

[A] White Bread

[B] Raw Vegetables

[C] Mashed Potatoes

[D] Grilled Fish

120. Which of the following conditions increases the risk of developing deep vein thrombosis (DVT)?

[A] Smoking
[B] Hypertension
[C] Obesity
[D] Hypoglycemia

121. Which comment by a friend indicates that a person is not processing their grief healthily after a loss?

[A] "I haven't cried at all since the funeral; it's as if nothing happened"
[B] "I'm still overwhelmed with sadness thinking about them every day"
[C] "I often find myself reminiscing about the good times we had together"
[D] "I've started talking about my feelings and seeking support from others"

122. What is a critical emergency situation that can arise from poorly managed diabetes mellitus?

[A] Hyperglycemia
[B] Ketoacidosis
[C] Gestational diabetes
[D] Chronic kidney disease

123. When managing a patient in labor with signs of fetal distress, which action is appropriate to take?

[A] Administer medications to induce labor
[B] Limit maternal position changes
[C] Increase maternal fluid intake
[D] Encourage the mother to push

124. What symptom is least likely to be associated with a patient having laryngeal cancer?

[A] Chronic cough
[B] Hoarseness
[C] Nausea and vomiting
[D] Sore throat

125. When is it appropriate to remove sutures after a surgical procedure?

[A] 7 to 10 days if healing is considered adequate
[B] 10 to 14 days regardless of healing
[C] 7 to 10 days only if there is no infection
[D] 14 to 21 days if the patient is stable

126. Which term refers to the process of the cervical tissue becoming thinner and softer in preparation for childbirth?

[A] Dilation

[B] Hyperplasia

[C] Effacement

[D] Symphysis

127. What should the nurse do if they observe a staff member handling the belongings of a patient without permission?

[A] Report the behavior to the charge nurse

[B] Confront the staff member directly

[C] Wait to see if items are reported missing

[D] Alert other staff members to keep an eye on the situation

128. In which fluid compartment is potassium primarily found?

[A] Intracellular fluid

[B] Plasma

[C] Extracellular fluid

[D] Lymphatic fluid

129. What is a primary objective of implementing quality assurance programs in healthcare?

[A] To provide financial incentives for staff

[B] To improve patient satisfaction scores

[C] To enhance patient safety and care quality

[D] To meet accreditation requirements

130. What is the primary treatment option for a patient diagnosed with giant cell arteritis?

[A] Ibuprofen

[B] Corticosteroids

[C] Anticoagulants

[D] High doses of prednisone

131. In which scenario should a nursing student seek clarification from a supervising nurse?

[A] The student uses a new blood pressure cuff properly

[B] The student does not perform hand hygiene before a patient assessment

[C] The student confirms the patient's identity before giving medication

[D] The student observes sterile techniques during a procedure

132. Which scenario illustrates a patient exercising their right to make an informed decision regarding their treatment?

[A] A patient declines a flu shot due to a belief in natural remedies

[B] A 45-year-old woman refuses chemotherapy after discussing the risks and benefits with her oncologist

[C] A minor signs a consent form for a medical procedure because their parent is unavailable

[D] An elderly man chooses to accept all recommended treatments without question

133. What dysrhythmia is the nurse most likely to encounter in a patient undergoing suctioning, indicating a possible decrease in heart rate?

[A] Bradycardia

[B] Ventricular tachycardia

[C] Atrial flutter

[D] Sinus tachycardia

134. What is the appropriate action for a client taking risedronate (Actonel) for osteoporosis?

[A] Lie down for at least 30 minutes after taking the medication

[B] Take the medication with food for better absorption

[C] Skip a dose if unable to take it in the morning

[D] Take the medication with a full glass of plain water and remain upright for 30 minutes

135. In terms of the affected areas of the gastrointestinal tract, which statement is true?

[A] Ulcerative colitis can affect the entire colon

[B] Crohn's disease can affect any part of the gastrointestinal tract

[C] Both conditions only affect the small intestine

[D] Ulcerative colitis only affects the small intestine

136. Which of the following describes the stages of an infectious process in the correct order?

[A] The inflammation, resolution, and healing stages

[B] The onset, progression, and recovery stages

[C] The incubation, prodromal, acute, and convalescence stages

[D] The incubation, prodromal, illness, and convalescence stages

137. Which monitoring pattern may suggest uteroplacental insufficiency?

[A] Bradycardia

[B] Tachycardia

[C] Variable decelerations

[D] Late decelerations

138. Which complication is associated with primary open-angle glaucoma?

[A] Loss of peripheral vision

[B] Severe eye pain

[C] Nausea and vomiting

[D] Sudden visual disturbances

139. What is the primary purpose of root cause analysis in quality improvement?

[A] To identify the underlying causes of problems

[B] To evaluate staff performance

[C] To create patient satisfaction surveys

[D] To implement new technology

140. When advising a patient with diverticulitis on food choices, which item is best to avoid?

[A] Cooked carrots

[B] Potato chips

[C] Bananas

[D] Nuts

141. Which condition should be closely monitored in a patient with potential hyperphosphatemia?

[A] Hypertension

[B] Anemia

[C] Coronary artery disease

[D] Chronic kidney disease

142. A patient presents with a potassium level of 8.0 mEq/L. Which treatment is most appropriate?

[A] Administer sodium bicarbonate

[B] Order intravenous calcium

[C] Increase dietary potassium

[D] Prepare for renal replacement therapy

143. What is the best nursing intervention to promote bilirubin excretion in an infant with jaundice?

[A] Encourage frequent feedings to promote hydration

[B] Limit the infant's exposure to light

[C] Reduce the infant's activity level

[D] Provide high-protein formulas

144. What are the characteristic features of Tetralogy of Fallot?

[A] Pulmonary stenosis, an atrial septal defect, right ventricular hypertrophy, and an overriding aorta

[B] Sub-aortic septal defect, an overriding aorta, right ventricular hypertrophy, and right ventricular outflow

[C] Ventricular septal defect, coarctation of the aorta, left ventricular hypertrophy, and an overriding aorta

[D] Ventricular septal defect, right ventricular hypertrophy, pulmonary stenosis, and an overriding aorta

145. What term is used to describe the condition of experiencing multiple miscarriages in successive pregnancies?

[A] Inevitable

[B] Missed

[C] Habitual

[D] Septic

146. A patient diagnosed with hypertension is advised to follow a low-sodium diet. Which of the following snacks would be appropriate for this patient?

[A] Salted nuts

[B] Potato chips

[C] Raw vegetables with hummus

[D] Processed cheese slices

147. After a lobectomy, what is the most common intervention to manage fluid accumulation in the pleural space?

[A] Administering bronchodilators

[B] Inserting a chest tube

[C] Providing supplemental oxygen

[D] Encouraging deep breathing exercises

148. When a nurse notices that the amount of a scheduled medication does not match with the records, which action should they prioritize?

[A] Notify the nursing supervisor

[B] Call the pharmacy department

[C] Send an email to the director of nursing

[D] Discuss the issue in the next team meeting

149. Which statement from the client indicates the need for additional support after being diagnosed with diabetes?

[A] I will ask for help with my meals

[B] I have difficulty understanding my medication schedule

[C] I can take care of my own feet

[D] I attend a diabetes support group

150. What is the average weight gain for infants during the first 4 months?

[A] 2 to 4 ounces per week

[B] 3 to 5 ounces per week

[C] 4 to 6 ounces per week

[D] 5 to 7 ounces per week

Answers

1. **A** – Protein intake is crucial after surgery to promote healing and maintain muscle mass, making it the most critical dietary component.
2. **B** – Furosemide (Lasix) IV must be administered cautiously and precisely, especially in clients with severe hypertension. The recommended practice is to use an infusion pump to carefully regulate the rate of administration and to ensure accurate dosing.
3. **D** – Thicker food textures can slow down swallowing and make it safer for clients with swallow difficulties.
4. **A** – Identifying oneself as a licensed nurse without the proper credentials misleads the public and can constitute fraud.
5. **B** – Administering furosemide at a rate of approximately 1 mL per minute helps prevent hypotension and other adverse effects.
6. **D** – A plasma phenytoin level of 25 mcg/mL exceeds the therapeutic range, indicating potential toxicity and requiring further evaluation.
7. **C** – Supportive family interactions are crucial as they foster trust and security in the infant, influencing emotional health and development positively.
8. **B** – Handling the tooth at the crown helps to protect the periodontal ligaments, which are crucial for reattachment.
9. **C** – Second degree burns affect the dermis, leading to pain and blistering due to intact pain receptors.

10. D – Respiratory distress signals possible airway compromise, tension pneumothorax, malposition or occlusion of the chest tube, or new bleeding—any of which can deteriorate within minutes.

11. B – Sodium is the primary electrolyte that regulates fluid balance, making it vital for maintaining proper hydration and blood volume.

12. C – Washing hands before and after caring for the cord is crucial to prevent infection and promote healing.

13. A – First, determine the hourly rate (800 cc / 6 hours = approximately 133.33 cc/hr). Calculate drops per minute: (133.33 cc/hr ÷ 60 min/hr) x 10 gtts/cc = approximately 22.2 gtts/min.

14. B – Tucking the chin towards the chest helps to close the airway and reduce the risk of aspiration.

15. C – Ball squeezing exercises are low-impact and aid in early rehabilitation by encouraging mobility and decreasing swelling.

16. A – Uric acid levels are primarily associated with gout, a condition characterized by high uric acid levels leading to joint inflammation.

17. D – Women over 35 are more likely to conceive twins due to hormonal changes that can lead to the release of more than one egg during ovulation.

18. C – Clients with sealed radioactive implants pose a risk for radiation exposure and should not be assigned to a pregnant nurse.

19. D – Hepatoblastoma is a liver cancer commonly seen in young children, distinguishing it from other types of cancers.

20. C – Liver disease often causes dry, itchy skin due to bile salt buildup. Fragrance-free moisturizers soothe the skin and prevent irritation. Hot water worsens pruritus, and sun exposure is not therapeutic here.

21. A – Women with breast implants can (and should) still have routine mammography, but the technologist must use implant-displacement (Eklund) views or similar modifications so that breast tissue is pulled forward and imaged separately from the implant.

22. D – Cushing's syndrome is characterized by excessive levels of cortisol, which is produced by the adrenal glands.

23. A – Ball-and-socket joints, like the shoulder, permit rotational movement and extensive range of motion.

24. **B** – Administering IV fluids is crucial in managing pancreatitis to ensure hydration and electrolyte balance.

25. **C** – The client with hypothyroidism would have a less demanding condition and is generally quieter, making them a suitable roommate for someone with myasthenia gravis.

26. **A** – Menopause is defined as the time when a woman has not experienced a menstrual period for 12 consecutive months, indicating the end of her reproductive years.

27. **B** – Tetralogy of Fallot consists of four specific heart defects: ventricular septal defect, right ventricular outflow tract obstruction, right ventricular hypertrophy, and an overriding aorta.

28. **D** – Lidocaine is specifically indicated for ventricular tachycardia as it reduces the rate of electrical impulses in the heart's ventricles.

29. **B** – Stridor is a high-pitched sound indicating upper airway obstruction, which is a critical respiratory concern.

30. **D** – Coma signifies severe impairment of neurological function often due to ammonia accumulation in patients with liver dysfunction.

31. **B** – Unexplained vaginal bleeding is a significant symptom that warrants reevaluation of hormone replacement therapy due to potential underlying issues.

32. **C** – Severe headaches are not generally produced by a primary laryngeal lesion and would prompt the nurse to consider an unrelated problem (e.g., migraine, hypertension) or distant metastatic disease, rather than the laryngeal cancer itself.

33. **A** – Cloudy dialysate may indicate infection, requiring laboratory analysis.

34. **C** – Serosanguineous is the term used for a type of exudate that is thin, red, and consists of serum mixed with blood, commonly observed in wound healing.

35. **A** – A soft stuffed animal is safe and encourages nurturing behaviors, suitable for this age group's developmental needs.

36. **B** – Mineral oil helps moisturize the skin and reduce itching, making it a suitable intervention for dry, irritated skin associated with hepatic conditions.

37. **B** – Evaluating the presence of peripheral pulse is essential to ensure adequate circulation, especially in patients with vascular concerns.

38. **C** – AST levels can elevate due to liver or muscle disease, making it less specific for heart damage.

39. **C** – A mosquito is a known vector that can transmit diseases like malaria and dengue fever to humans.

40. A – Antivert (meclizine) is an antihistamine that helps alleviate vertigo symptoms associated with Meniere's disease.

41. A – Breast implants can obscure the breast tissue, making it difficult to detect abnormalities during a mammogram.

42. D – Alopecia, or hair loss, is a common side effect of many chemotherapeutic agents and significantly impacts a patient's self-image.

43. B – Cleft palate surgery is typically performed before 12 months to support better language development and growth.

44. C – Airborne transmission requires a negative pressure room to prevent the spread of infectious agents.

45. C – Selecting a dressing that is suitable for the type of wound is crucial in preventing moisture-related skin damage.

46. D – Mammograms are the standard imaging test used to detect breast tumors and other anomalies, providing essential information for diagnosis.

47. A – Cachexia is specifically linked to chronic diseases and is marked by significant weight loss and muscle mass decrease.

48. D – Lactulose works by reducing ammonia absorption in the intestines, helping to alleviate symptoms of hepatic encephalopathy.

49. C – Duchenne's muscular dystrophy leads to gradual muscle degeneration and may be confused with normal developmental stages, making early recognition crucial.

50. C – The surgeon is the appropriate person to clarify the surgical procedure and its risks, adhering to the principle of informed consent.

51. B – Saliva substitutes are specifically designed to relieve dryness of the mouth and are the most effective choice.

52. B – The incubation stage precedes the prodromal stage, followed by the illness stage, and concludes with the convalescence stage in the infection process.

53. A – Increasing hydration is key in promoting the elimination of bilirubin from the infant's system.

54. C – Cephalohematoma is specifically located outside the cranium and beneath the periosteum, not crossing suture lines.

55. D – Hypokalemia is indicated by the critically low potassium level of 2.5 mEq/L.

56. A – Full-term infants typically require 120 calories per kilogram to support their growth.

57. **D** – Performing hand hygiene regularly is proven to be the most effective method to reduce the risk of infections in healthcare settings.

58. **A** – Psychosocial risk factors encompass behaviors and lifestyle choices including substance use and mental health conditions.

59. **B** – Prolonged lactation can lead to calcium depletion from bones, increasing the risk of osteoporosis in women.

60. **A** – Biofeedback is crucial for providing patients with real-time feedback on their bodily functions, enabling them to learn self-regulation of emotions and stress.

61. **B** – Monitoring blood glucose is critical while on TPN since the solution is rich in carbohydrates and may cause elevated glucose levels.

62. **A** – Vesicular breath sounds are characteristic of healthy lungs, while the other options are associated with respiratory distress.

63. **A** – Immobility causes a negative nitrogen balance due to muscle breakdown and decreased protein synthesis.

64. **B** – Erik Erikson is recognized for his eight stages of psychosocial development, each associated with a specific conflict that must be resolved.

65. **C** – The correct action involves documenting the incident thoroughly and issuing a reprimand to address the issue while allowing for improvement.

66. **C** – Discussing the behavior privately allows for direct communication and potential resolution while maintaining professionalism.

67. **D** – Covering the exposed organs with a sterile saline-soaked dressing helps to keep the tissue moist and protected until further medical assistance is available.

68. **A** – Passing the NCLEX-PN examination demonstrates the necessary knowledge and skills required to ensure safe patient care.

69. **C** – Prolonged immobility, such as sitting for long periods during travel or after surgery, increases the risk of DVT due to lack of movement in the lower extremities.

70. **D** – An infant's skull is composed of 6 bones: 2 frontal, 2 parietal, 1 occipital, and 1 ethmoid. These bones are connected by sutures and fontanelles that allow for brain growth.

71. **A** – Comatose is the least responsive level of consciousness, where the individual shows no response to external stimuli.

72. **B** – Advance directives detail the patient's preferences regarding medical interventions, including the refusal of specific treatments.

73. B – A bivalve cast helps accommodate swelling, preventing increased pressure and associated complications.

74. C – The Parkland Formula is specifically designed to calculate the amount of fluid required for burn patients based on their body weight and the extent of their burns.

75. D – A power outage disrupts the normal operation of a healthcare facility and poses risks to patient safety, thus it is categorized as an internal disaster.

76. B – The client with asthma showing signs of wheezing may be experiencing an acute exacerbation, needing urgent assessment.

77. A – AST is not specific to myocardial injury and can be elevated in various other conditions.

78. C – Newborns commonly lose weight initially as a result of normal physiological processes including loss of fluid and expulsion of meconium.

79. B – The nurse in answer B has the relevant obstetric experience needed to recognize and manage hypertension in postpartum clients.

80. D – Respiratory distress indicates potential life-threatening issues that require urgent attention.

81. D – Saturated fats can raise LDL cholesterol levels, so patients with hyperlipidemia should limit their intake.

82. A – Failure to follow a physician's orders for a critical patient can lead to severe consequences for the patient's health and must be reported to the Board.

83. C – Alert is the most responsive state of consciousness, followed by confused, lethargic, obtunded, stuporous, and comatose.

84. C – Stage III is the surgical stage where patients are adequately anesthetized and do not respond to surgical stimuli.

85. D – Drug tolerance is the body's reduced response to a drug after prolonged use, requiring increased dosages for effective pain management.

86. D – Appendicitis is most common in teenagers and individuals in their early 20s, making them the demographic at highest risk.

87. C – Squeezing a soft ball promotes circulation and helps regain strength in the arm and shoulder after a mastectomy.

88. C – A brain tumor can lead to increased intracranial pressure due to mass effect, resulting in papilledema.

89. A – There are 16 minims in 1 milliliter, multiplying by 5 gives you 80 minims in 5 milliliters.

90. D – Changes in family dynamics can significantly impact an infant's psychosocial development as they perceive their caregivers' responses and stressors associated with their chronic condition.

91. C – The classic risk factors for gallstones follow the "Four F's": Female, Forty, Fertile, and Fat. Hispanic women, especially around age 40, have a higher prevalence due to genetic and hormonal factors.

92. B – Adjuvant medications are designed to enhance the effects of primary analgesics, making them more effective in pain management.

93. D – Vesicular breath sounds are a sign of normal lung function, whereas the other options indicate abnormalities.

94. B – Diabetes insipidus is characterized by insufficient ADH, resulting in excessive thirst and urination.

95. A – Stage IV pressure ulcers are noted for deep tissue damage and may show exposure of bone, muscle, or tendons, indicating a severe level of tissue injury.

96. C – An appropriate expected outcome should be specific and measurable, such as rating pain, which identifies a clear target for pain management.

97. B – The nurse's response shows respect for the client's beliefs and supports their emotional needs during a medical procedure.

98. B – An LPN is not authorized to initiate a blood transfusion; this is a responsibility of a registered nurse.

99. B – Calcium and vitamin D are essential for bone health and reducing the risk of fractures in clients with osteoporosis.

100. A – The apical pulse assessment involves listening to the heart for rate and irregularities, which is crucial for identifying arrhythmias.

101. B – Prolactin is essential for milk production after childbirth, while other hormones play different roles in the reproductive system.

102. C – Bathe the deceased patient using standard precautions to prevent any risk of infection transmission.

103. B – The 28-year-old female experiencing a manic episode would benefit most from admission to a medical unit specializing in mental health, as she requires specialized psychiatric care.

104. D – Dilation refers specifically to the process of the cervix opening to allow for the passage of the baby during labor.

105. C – Osgood-Schlatter disease is characterized by inflammation of the patellar tendon, often due to repetitive stress from sports.

106. A – Dorothea Orem created the Self-Care Deficit Theory, emphasizing patients' abilities to perform self-care.

107. D – Adequate hydration and fiber intake are critical for effective bowel function during pregnancy.

108. C – Perimenopause is characterized by hormonal fluctuations leading to symptoms such as hot flashes and mood changes before menstrual periods cease.

109. B – A greenstick fracture is an incomplete fracture that bends the bone, frequently observed in children due to their softer, more flexible bones.

110. B – Lawrence Kohlberg is known for his theory of moral development, outlining the stages individuals go through in their understanding of morality.

111. D – Urinalysis is a key part of prenatal care to check for issues like preeclampsia and diabetes.

112. B – An episiotomy is a surgical procedure that involves making an incision in the perineum to assist in the delivery process.

113. A – The presence of an indwelling urinary catheter is a known risk factor for acquiring a healthcare-associated infection during hospitalization.

114. D – Clear nasal drainage could indicate cerebrospinal fluid leakage, which requires urgent assessment and intervention.

115. A – Patients with an ICD should avoid using electronic devices like cellphones on the side of the device to prevent interference.

116. A – ABCDE helps identify significant health concerns such as allergies, bleeding risks, cortisone use, diabetes management, and history of embolic events.

117. D – The embryonic period lasts until the end of the 12th week, encompassing critical development stages.

118. A – Evidence-based practice integrates clinical expertise and patient preferences with the best available evidence to optimize patient care.

119. B – Clients with diverticulitis should eliminate gas-forming foods like raw vegetables to prevent abdominal pain.

120. C – Obesity is a well-known risk factor for DVT due to its association with prolonged venous stasis and increased pressure in the venous system.

121. A – The statement shows a lack of emotional processing and could indicate suppressed grief.

122. B – Ketoacidosis is a serious condition that can occur when the body starts breaking down fats at an excessive rate due to lack of insulin, leading to high levels of ketones in the blood.

123. C – Increasing maternal fluid intake can help support fetal circulation and reduce distress symptoms.

124. C – Nausea and vomiting are not typical symptoms of laryngeal cancer, whereas the other options are more commonly reported.

125. A – Sutures can generally be removed in 7 to 10 days if the surgical site shows adequate healing.

126. C – Effacement is the specific term used to describe the softening and thinning of the cervix, which occurs as labor progresses.

127. A – Reporting the behavior to the charge nurse ensures that the appropriate steps can be taken to investigate and address the violation of patient privacy.

128. A – Potassium is mainly located in the intracellular fluid, while sodium and chloride dominate the extracellular fluid.

129. C – Quality assurance programs focus on enhancing patient safety and the quality of care provided, which directly impacts patient outcomes.

130. D – High doses of prednisone are effective in reducing inflammation associated with giant cell arteritis.

131. B – Not performing hand hygiene before any patient interaction increases the risk of infection.

132. B – Informed decision-making involves the patient understanding and considering the risks and benefits of a treatment, which the 45-year-old woman does after discussing with her doctor.

133. A – Bradycardia may occur during suctioning due to stimulation of the vagus nerve.

134. D – Actonel should be taken with a full glass of water, and the client should remain upright to reduce the risk of esophageal irritation.

135. B – Crohn's disease can affect any segment of the gastrointestinal tract, while ulcerative colitis is limited to the colon.

136. D – The incubation, prodromal, illness, and convalescence stages represent the recognized phases of how an infection develops and resolves.

137. D – Late decelerations typically occur due to impaired placental perfusion or uteroplacental insufficiency.

138. A – Primary open-angle glaucoma often leads to gradual loss of peripheral vision without the acute symptoms found in angle-closure glaucoma.

139. A – Root cause analysis aims to uncover the fundamental issues leading to problems, ensuring that solutions address the root rather than just surface-level symptoms.

140. D – Nuts can be problematic due to their hard texture and potential for seeds.

141. D – Chronic kidney disease can lead to phosphate retention, increasing the risk of hyperphosphatemia.

142. B – Intravenous calcium helps stabilize the heart's electrical activity in case of high potassium levels, and is a critical initial treatment.

143. A – Frequent feedings help in increasing hydration, thereby promoting bilirubin excretion through urine.

144. D – The four classic components of Tetralogy of Fallot are: Ventricular septal defect (VSD), Right ventricular hypertrophy, Pulmonary stenosis, Overriding aorta. Option [D] is the only one that correctly includes all four.

145. C – Habitual abortion refers specifically to three or more consecutive miscarriages, indicating a pattern of loss.

146. C – Raw vegetables with hummus are low in sodium and suitable for a low-sodium diet.

147. B – A chest tube is used post-operatively to drain air, blood, or fluid from the pleural space, which is essential after lung surgery.

148. A – The nursing supervisor is the appropriate contact for immediate reporting of medication discrepancies, ensuring quick resolution.

149. B – Difficulty understanding medication schedules suggests the client may not manage their diabetes effectively, necessitating follow-up education.

150. D – Newborns typically gain about 5 to 7 ounces per week during the first few months of life, reflecting healthy growth.

ACCESS NCLEX-PN ONLINE RESOURCES

Congratulations on reaching the end of the book!

We hope this guide has helped you prepare for your NCLEX-PN exam, but your study journey doesn't stop here! To further support your success, we've included exclusive study tools:

- **Test Simulator** – Generate unlimited NCLEX-PN-style practice tests from a pool of 700+ questions to reinforce your knowledge.
- **Digital Flashcards** – Reinforce key nursing concepts with interactive flashcards for effective learning.
- **Printable Case Scenarios** – Practice clinical judgment with real-world nursing scenarios for each chapter.
- **SYSTEM-14 & Mindshift Course** – Learn a proven method to master content efficiently and build the right mindset for exam success.

These resources are completely free and available to you for life. To access them, simply visit the URL below or scan the QR code with your device. Then, enter the code **nclexpn2829** when prompted for access.

Thank you for choosing this book. We wish you great success on your exam!

tinyurl.com/msp-nclexpn

Access code: **nclexpn2829**